Physician
S**U**rgeon
Tu**B**erculosis
Scar**L**et Fever
Mend**I**cant
Va**C**cinator

St Ant**H**ony's Fire
M**E**asles
Dise**A**se
I**L**lness
Doc**T**or
Dyn **H**ysbys

Peter Ford retired after 45 years in the NHS to live in mid Wales. Here he developed a keen interest in local history, and become a town guide. His passion is to tell the often forgotten stories of local people. To explore the lives of those who suffered misfortune or oppression, and about whom myths and legends have arisen. Where did these come from and is there any truth in them?

Also by Peter Ford
The Tragic Lives Series.

Tragic Lives 2
Mary Morgan.
Victim or Villain of 18th Century Infanticide.

Tragic Lives 3
Fair Rosamund
Mistress of King Henry II.

Available from Amazon.

Doctors, Disease, and Death.

The Story of Public Health in Hay on Wye.

Peter Ford

Amazon Paperback.
Copyright © Peter Charles Ford.
First published in Great Britain in 2021.
Peter Charles Ford has asserted his right to be asserted as the author of this work in accordance with the Copyright, Design and Patents Act 1988.

All rights reserved.
No part of this publication may be reproduced, stored in a retrieval system, or transmitted, in any form or by any means without the prior written permission of the publisher, nor be otherwise circulated in any form of binding or cover other than that in which it is published and without a similar condition being imposed on any subsequent purchaser.

Dedication

To my wife Angela.
Your help and support made this book possible.

Acknowledgements

For the story of The Home Visit I am indebted to Mrs Janet Robinson.

For the extensive information on Rosa Blanche Williams I am grateful for the assistance provided by Mrs Marion Lally, the daughter of Rosa's youngest child Richard Allan Williams. She is one of Rosa's 19 grandchildren.

While I have not met Mrs Joan Barnes I have her to thank for recording the eye-witness reminiscences of her father Constable Bailey, Christmas 1988. Interview CD courtesy of Mrs Mari Fforde.

Contents

The Home Visit	1
Chapter 1 – Medieval Medicine	5
Chapter 2 – Disease	29
Chapter 3 – Emergency Medicine	57
Chapter 4 – Public Health	75
Chapter 5 – Clinical Services	102
Chapter 6 – Medical Services	141
Appendix 1: Rosa Blanche Williams	209
Appendix 2: Alice Agnes de Winton	219
References	228

Old Hay Superstition.

> *'Never pay your doctor's bill in full,
> or you are shortly going to need his services again.'*

The Home Visit

"A farmer's wife had requested a home visit and she suggested that while I was there I might go on up the hill and call on her neighbours, old J. and his wife. She said she was worried about them. Well, I hadn't been up there for about fifteen years and to tell you the truth if someone had asked me about them, I'd have said they were probably dead. But I took their notes with me and, having the rest of the morning, I went up the track and found the little house tucked into the side of the hill, almost in a little ravine. I have to say I haven't enjoyed a visit so much for years. It was marvellous.

J. and his wife are two lovely old souls and they gave me a real welcome. Their kitchen was pure nineteenth century. There were lots of cats, no electricity, no piped water – just a stream running outside the back door – and there was an earth closet outside. It was very dark inside because several of the windows had broken and they were covered with pieces of cardboard.

> 'I hear you're not well, J.'
> 'Well,' he said. 'I've got a bit of a pain round here.' And he indicated his chest.
> 'Do you get it often?'
> 'A bit.'
> 'Have you had it long?'
> He thought: 'A fair bit.'
> 'And does it hurt much?'
> 'A bit.'

Now, wherever you go outside that cottage its always uphill. Either you go straight up from the back door to the skyline, or about twenty yards on the other side and then straight up. Wondering if J.'s heart was the problem, I asked him if he'd been outside much.

> 'I've been up the hill to sheep – twice,' he said, waving an arm towards the far top of the hill.
> 'When?'
> 'This morning.'
> 'What twice?'
> 'Ay.'
> 'And how old are you, J?'
> 'Eighty-seven.'

I decided it couldn't be his heart so I tried a new tack.

> 'Do you ever get the pain when you've eaten something?'
> 'Sometimes.'
> 'What do you like to eat?'

I could see that they couldn't cook much because they only had a big open fire with a grill above it where an old iron kettle was bubbling away.

'I like bread and cheese,' he said after due thought.

'Does that give you the pain?'

'A bit.'

'Has it stopped you eating it?'

'Sometimes.'

'Have you ever been sick?'

'A bit.'

'What colour is it?'

'Ordinary.'

'Well, is it red, black or yellowish?'

'No, just ordinary.'

'When were you sick?'

'A bit ago.'

'Well, yesterday?'

'No.'

'Well, last week?'

He shook his head and looked questioningly at his wife, then suggested 'Ah, it was after I came out of hospital.'

I was surprised because I thought I would have known about a hospital visit. I tried to look at his notes – such a thin folder – but I had to go outside because it was too dark in the kitchen, even though it was only the middle of the morning. I couldn't see any mention of hospital so I went back in.

'How long ago were you in hospital?'
He shook his head, puzzled. 'A bit.'
'I know when it was,' broke in his wife. 'It was just after your mother died, J.'
'Ay, so it was.'
'So when was that?' I asked.
'1947.'

This was 25 years previously so at that point I gave up but suggested that the next time their neighbour brought them down into Hay he should come to the surgery.

I dropped in on their neighbour on my way down and she said she'd bring them on market day. 'They're terrified, you know,' she said. 'Terrified that someone will try to move them down to the village. It'd kill them, of course.' "

This incident may have been first related thirty years ago, and occurred in the 1970's, but it could have occurred almost any time over the last two centuries. And it is true.

Perhaps it is not typical, but probably not a totally unique incident for a rural doctor working in an isolated small market town in the Marches. Dealing with independent country folk reluctant to trouble the doctor would always be a challenge.

Go back another century, before antibiotics and fully equipped hospitals were there as a backup, and medical practice would have presented even greater challenges.

.

Chapter 1 – Medieval Medicine

In our modern wealthy society with its free state funded healthcare it is easy to forget just how perilous life was for people years ago. Covid 19 may not have been a problem, but there were any number of other highly infectious contagious diseases. These spread through families like wildfire. And it was not just the dangers of disease. Scant regard for health and safety meant serious accidental injury was very common.

There were no effective drugs to treat disease. Medical care to alleviate pain or to lessen life changing deformity from broken bones was very basic. Illness and accidents, and the consequences of them, were perils of normal everyday life, and there were limited places to turn for help when you became ill.

The Middle Ages was a time of strong religious belief, and anyone who became ill would first and foremost seek spiritual help from their local church. Doing pilgrimage to a famous shrine was popular. It was often only as a last resort that help might be sought from a local healer, and this after the priest had been called.

As the power of religion declined superstition became more prominent in rural beliefs. Typical of this was the experience of the famous curate of Clyro. The Rev. Francis Kilvert visited Mr and Mrs Meredith on his rounds on the 8 August 1878. They were old country folk. Mrs Meredith said she was ill, and predicted that she would not be better until the passing of the evil dog star in three days' time.

On another occasion a friend of Kilverts, Miss Thomas, recounted that a wheelwright from Llanigon, a Mr Phillips, charmed away Alice Lewis' toothache. He did it by giving her a 65-word religious charm to be worn around her neck. How big this item was we do not know. It may have been religious, and 'cured' her toothache, but it had more in keeping with medieval religious belief and superstition than medical practice.

People would have relied heavily on traditional folk medicines, and the remedies of the Dyn Hysbys – the cunning men. Much of their knowledge would have been permeating through the countryside for centuries, although it should not be thought that it was all country folklore and magic healing.[1]

Historically Wales has not been a backwater as far as the medicial practice of the time is concerned. In fact it has a long history of being at the forefront of medicine going back to at least 1000 BC. By 430BC the laws of the Cornish King Dynwal Moelmud covered the art of medicine, and provided an element of state protection. These laws were based on mysticism combined with herbal remedies.

Knowledge of them spread to Wales through the activities of Druids and Ovates, who were kinds of seers and herbalists. Their practice shows evidence of Greek influence, possibly due to trade links, and the work of Hippocrates, the Father of Medicine, was highly rated.

A significant milestone in Welsh healing arts was the so-called Laws of Howel Dda king of Dyfed from AD 942-948. He set down a code of laws that continued to be used by the Welsh until the time of Edward I.

One of these related to the office of Physician to the Royal Court. It defined a list of duties and appropriate conduct, but in return the incumbent was provided with land, clothes and a horse by the crown. When in the palace his duties were to be given to all freely. While he could not leave the court without the king's permission, when he was out and about he was under the king's protection. A scale of fees for his services was also laid down.

The Laws of Howel Dda prevailed until around AD1200. At that time King Rhys Grug (Rhys the hoarse or stammerer) had a physician Rhiwallon who living in Myddfai Carmarthenshire with his three sons. The family began a collection of cures and remedies for various diseases, recording them in a manuscript for the first time. A copy of this record is still available today in the British Museum, and a part copy, The Red Book, is in Jesus College Oxford.

The story of these famous healers and the legend of the Physicians of Myddfai, only 40 miles from Hay, is well known. Accounts of the source of their mystical powers is common to many cultures, although details differ. In Wales these relate to a Lady and the lake of Llyn-y-Fan Fach on the northern slopes of the Black Mountains in Carmarthenshire.

The legend speaks of a beautiful woman who emerges from a lake, and a passing widow's son. He falls in love with her and persuades her to marry him but is given a warning. If he should strike her three times, even accidentally, she will disappear back into the lake.

The couple live happily together, and have three sons, but over time inevitably the man accidentally strikes his wife three times. On the third occasion she disappears back into the lake, taking with her all their livestock.

Her sons are heartbroken and often wander by the lake. One day the lady appears to her eldest son. She gives him a bag of herbs and instructions on how to use them for healing. Her advice and knowledge allow the sons to build a core of medical treatments that makes them renowned healers.

The Physicians of Myddfai are mentioned in folk law from the 14th century. Their fame spread across South Wales, and they went on to practice throughout Wales. Their skills were passed from generation to generation until the last direct descendants died in 1739/43.

The physicians based their work on a good diet, modest lifestyle and herbal remedies. A typical remedy that may have some relevance today is:

"Whoever is fat, let him drink of the juice of fennel and it will reduce him."

Inevitably many of the remedies were for common conditions such as colds, coughs and sleeping potions. Analysis of the diseases they treated shows that eye and skin conditions were the most common, followed by wounds and broken bones, chest and throat problems, and such things as intestinal worms and kidney stones.

Most of the ailments are attributable to lifestyle and living conditions. Broken bones and wounds were caused by accidents or perhaps the violent nature of the times. Eye disease could be the consequence of living with smoky fires. The general lack of hygiene encouraged worms. Damp conditions would account for chest disease. There is little mention of heart disease, strokes or degenerative ailments.

The remedies on which their healing was based used the whole of a herb rather than one active ingredient. It is this use of the multitude of properties within a herb to treat the whole body which may have been the key to their success. A similar philosophy is followed in modern herbalism.

The physicians also defined the personal qualities of a good practitioner and need for a duty of care to patients. James Davis 1648–1722 wrote his Book of Iago ap Dewi which listed a number of medical maxims which still apply today. 'Moderate exercise is health', 'Better is appetite than gluttony', 'A dry cough is the trumpet of death'.

Notwithstanding their fame the Physicians of Myddfai were not the only Welsh healers. Bened Feddyg from the Vale of Clywd wrote a medical manuscript which was added to through four generations of his family.[2]

During the 15th century there were a number of important medical treaties written in Wales. The Book of Talgarth, the village near Hay, contained a manuscript known as Havod 16. This listed numerous herbs for medicinal use. It is thought that many could have been grown by the monks at Llantony Abbey in the Black Mountains just 11 miles from Hay.

Although not born in Wales Thomas Phaer 1510-1560 lived most of his life in Pembrokeshire. His Boke of Childryn on the care of the very young led to him being regarded as the father of paediatrics.

These medieval physicians built their practices on traditional herbal remedies, and a basic knowledge of many of these would have been commonplace. As a consequence the division between physicians and the local wise women in many cases would have been ill defined, although it is to be hoped that physicians were less liable to use treatments based only on folklore, superstition or old wives tales.

Herbal Medicine.

Inevitably the few physicians there were would have lived at a distance from much of the rural population. This made it awkward and inconvenient to visit them, and expensive to call them out.

In such circumstances members of the gentry would occasionally be able to help. Many acquired basic medical skills in military service, particularly in the case of accidents. In other circumstances, and for those who preferred to put their trust in the old beliefs, the local wise woman would be consulted.

Typical country remedies could include:

- Fennel and mistletoe crushed and rubbed into the gum relieved toothache.
- Slices of giant puffball would be placed over open wounds to treat them. It was common for them to be collected before battles for just such a purpose. Alternatively they could be rubbed into a powder and used on wet sores or weeping wounds.
- Willow bark boiled for at least an hour made a very effective pain killer, the predecessor of modern-day aspirin.
- Garlic was used to treat typhoid fever and gastro-intestinal tract problems such as food poisoning and amoebic dysentery.
- Plantain added to washing water was effective against lice.
- Cider vinegar relieved kidney and bladder stones.
- Nettles boiled in water made a good hair shampoo, and a wineglassful three times a day was used to treat blood pressure.
- An ounce of rosemary boiled in one pint of water rubbed into the scalp made a good hair stimulant.
- Bathing twice daily in two pints of parsnip water and one teaspoon of powdered alum cured chilblains.
- Carrying the herb mugwort was said to combat tiredness.

- Asthma could be eased by the cooled liquid of one ounce of sweet chestnut leaves in one and a half pints of water to which was added half an ounce of honey and half an ounce of glycerine.

Rheumatism and sciatica were common rural ailments for which there were a number of treatments.

- Goose grease could be rubbed in.
- Cider vinegar would ease it.
- The cooled liquid of one ounce of ragwort boiled in one pint of water taken three times a day eased sciatica.
- An ounce of dandelion root boiled for 20 mins in one and a half pints of water drunk twice a day helped with rheumatic pains.

Some of these traditional cures have surprised modern researchers with their healing qualities. Recently a 10th century eye balm has been recreated from Bald's Leechbook, which is housed in the British Library. Leech was an old term for doctor.

The recipe uses 30g of crushed onion and the same of crushed garlic, mixed with 50ml of white wine and 50ml of cow's bile salts from their gallbladder. The mixture is then stored for nine days in the dark at 4C, and strained before use.

Laboratory tests have shown this eye balm is a very effective bacteria killer for ulcers and burns, surpassing antibiotics in some cases.[3] Previous research has already shown it is an effective treatment for the superbug Multi Resistant Staphylococcus Aureus (M.R.S.A.).

We do not know how widespread this, or any other creams, ointments, or medicines, were generally available. However there was one common substance which has been used from time immemorial to aid healing. From the time of the Egyptians, through the ancient Greeks and Romans, to the Middle Ages honey was used as an antiseptic agent.

It is currently making a strong comeback as modern science has rediscovered its powers for healing and its antibacterial properties. In this age of antibiotic resistant infection, it has been found effective to apply honey based wound care products routinely on patients following plastic surgery.[4]

Folklore and Superstition.

Folklore treatments tended to follow common lines, and many appear bizarre to modern eyes. Often they were worse than in Roman times. One 14th century remedy for quinsy (throat abscesses) involved killing a cat and stuffing it with bear and hedgehog grease mixed with herbs. This was roasted and the grease obtained rubbed into the skin.

Another attributed toothache to worms. This idea may have derived from The Legend of The Worm inscribed on a Babylonian cuneiform tablet. The legend described tooth worms drinking blood and eating the roots of teeth, possibly an allegory for infection but often taken literally until recent times.

Folklore described how placing a lighted candle on the tooth drew the worms out into a cup of water placed in the mouth![5] Often use of these and other 'treatments' was guided by astrological influences, such as the phases of the moon.

Practical remedies were usually in the hands of those with some anatomical knowledge, such as butchers. Gradually barbers took over the role and a current reminder of this is the barbers pole. Originally this would have been wound with red and white bandages to make the stripes. The brass bleeding bowl was then hung from the pole by a chain, although this became reduced to the brass cap over time.

Cauterising was common practice. Hot pokers were applied to a particular area of the body, and not just confined to the staunching of blood flow after a cut or injury.

Other practices such as wearing a magpie's beak around the neck to treat toothache, and cutting a hole in the skull (trepanning) to let the devil out and treat madness were little more than superstitious nonsense.

There were numerous other bizarre treatments, all equally ineffective, such as washing in a boy's urine to treat ringworm, covering a sore with a dead wolf's skin, eating ginger for loss of memory, eating treacle for loss of speech, spotty skin or snake bites, applying bacon fat mixed with wild boar grease to treat bruises, and the prevention of hangovers by drinking with your hat off to let the bad vapours out.

'Taking the waters' became fashionable in Georgian times but had existed for many years. The healing properties of the wellsprings around Llanwrtyd were well known, and there were many other local wells with properties said to cure such things as sprains or eye disease.

Water doctors who examined the urine of patients to decide their course of treatment continued to practice into the 18th and 19th centuries long after it was abandoned by conventional medicine.

By the early part of the 19th century medical practice was a combination of common sense, chance, and superstition. Bloodletting and the use of leeches were still common, together with laxatives, poultices and 'taking the waters'. Underpinning much of this was the continued reliance on botanical remedies.

Around this time a record of ancient cures and remedies was collected at Llangattock, just across the Black Mountains from Hay.

- A number of cures for pneumonia were allegedly successful following the killing a Pencroeslan sheep. The warm spleen was placed against the foot of the patient, right foot for the left lung and vice versa, and left for 24 hours. This was repeated for 3 days killing a fresh lamb each time. The spleen was removed when it was found to be wrinkled and smelled badly. On each occasion the patient was said to have recovered.
- Less successful was the treatment observed by Dr Morgan in 1925 when lamb's lungs were tied to the feet of a man desperately ill with pneumonia. Needless to say this did not prevent a fatal outcome.

- To remove a buried black thorn a sow's gallbladder would be applied to the puncture site, and then the thorn could be successful drawn.
- A number of remedies for the relief of whooping cough were recorded. To sooth violent coughing one wineglass of 'mouse broth' was taken. This was made by pouring 2 gallons of boiling water over a dead mouse and allowing it to cool. Other popular remedies to sooth the coughing were long brisk walks, entering a cave such as Llangattock cave or the Devils Arch, a tunnel under a canal, or having your head pushed out of a train window as it passed through a tunnel.
- A popular remedy for night cramps was to wrap copper wire around your ankles when going to bed.
- The use of cobwebs to heal cuts has long been a Romany treatment.
- Treatment for kidney disease might include giving the patient couch grass root tea.

Other well-known remedies included:

- Filling a milk bottle with boiling water, pour it out and immediately placing it over a boil. The resultant vacuum sucked the infected matter out. Methylated spirits lit in a bottle had a similar effect.
- Eel or adder skins were credited with treating rheumatism, blood poisoning and also facilitating the removal of foreign bodies buried beneath the skin.[6]

- The dead featured in a number of cures - the rope from a hanged man placed around the head cured headaches. The hand of a dead person, preferably a malefactor, cured 'wens' or sebaceous cysts beneath the skin.[7]
- There is a whole library of cures for warts - dipping your hand in a blacksmiths cooling tank, tying a horse-hair around it, rubbing it with a black snail, cutting a potato in half and throwing away one half while leaving the other to decay, rubbing with elderberry leaves picked at night and then burning them, etc. etc.
- Poultices were popular and might include bacon fat or bread and groundsel. The Rev. Francis Kilvert had a boil on his thigh treated by Dr Clouston 22nd April 1871 with 3 or 4 hourly linseed poultices.
- Snail water or snail milk distilled from crushed snail shells, ivy, and milk was given to patients two or three times a day for consumption i.e. tuberculosis. Other recipes added alcohol, balm, ox-eye daisies or even talcum powder.[8]

Amongst other medicines, including snail milk, kept in the housekeeper's cabinet at imposing Berrington Hall, near Leominster, was Oil of Earthworm. It was commonly known as Bruise Medicine.

Rubbing the feet of a baby in snow to prevent them ever getting chilblains was popular until recent times. London evacuee Edward Stapleton records being made to run barefoot in the snow down Church

Street in Hay in 1943 by his 'Auntie Kit' for this reason.[9]

Charmers.

Mendicants or wandering healers travelled through the towns and villages of the borderlands, but charmers would often be the first line of resort. They were more likely to be local and cheaper than other healers.

Certain individuals were credited with great power as charmers. Within walking distance of Hay John E. was a famous charmer in Weobley, but no doubt there were others. They had charms for burns, toothache, the ague (fevers), stopping bleeding, sprains, dog bites and various other maladies. Many remedies had a religious element invoked Jesus Christ or 'our Lord and Saviour', and sometimes the Virgin or Peter.

Cures recorded at Weobley, as well as elsewhere, included preventing cramp by wearing an eel skin gaiter around the lower leg. Placing the hairs of a donkey, or alternatively woodlice, in a bag around a baby's neck would alleviate teething problems. Mistletoe tea was believed to prevent fits, ground up pieces of hot cross bun taken in water treated tummy problems year-round, and the inner bark of an elder tree boiled in milk would treat jaundice.

A large number of 'cures' involved passing an object (thread, snail, bacon fat, bread) over an area then disposing of said object or allowing it to decay. As it did so the malady was cured.

Such a treatment for warts was to pass a white slug across it north to south and then east to west before impaling it on a thorn bush. Other charms included placing a wreath of ivy leaves around the scalp of someone with ringworm to cure it.

In April 1852 an unsuccessful instance of charming occurred at Peterchurch in the Golden Valley. It demonstrates how primitive the treatments were that people put their faith in.

An 11-year-old boy Charles James was working in a barn when he fell and hurt his foot and ankle. On the Thursday evening the pain was so bad he had to stop work and his leg swelled. By Monday he was in bed and 'Mrs Hadley had applied a vinegar and bran poultice'.

The following day it was even more painful, so he was taken to Mrs Matthews who was noted for her charming powers. She said the leg was not broken and getting on well with the poultices. As he did not improve on the Saturday evening he was taken to David Jenkins, a charmer. He changed the poultice to one with sheep's droppings which had been boiled.

By Tuesday Charles was worse and a surgeon, Mr Reece, saw him. He recommended a hot brick on his cold foot and left some medicine, but it was too late to save Charles. By the next morning he was dead. A verdict of death by natural causes was passed.[10]

While this might seem primitive even 'orthodox' medical treatment at the time was horrific by modern standards. The Rev. Francis Kilvert records on Friday 18 November 1870 he went to see young Meredith. His jaw had locked six months previously following an attack of mumps. The treatment at Hereford Infirmary had been unsuccessful when they tried to prise his jaws apart with a screw lever.

Another noted charmer was Solomon Chilton of Llanelly although he worked primarily with animals.

Healers.

Some individuals were credited with exceptional skills as healers as opposed to charmers. Often this would involve some form of massage or manipulation. Ted Lloyd was a highly regarded bone setter in Crickhowell until 1922. His practice was continued by his son and daughter until about 1948.

People would travel long distances to consult such people.

Bloodletting.

The practice of bloodletting by knife to remove bad blood from an affected area was a long-established medical practice. Popular from ancient times it was widely employed nationally up until the mid 1800's. It was thought to reduce the 'humours', and losses of ten or more pints over a number of days were not uncommon.

Medicinal leeches (*Hirudo medicinalis*) were also used for similar, if less extreme, purposes. Leech Pool is a 2.3-hectare shallow swampy pond near Clifford in the Wye valley. It may have derived its name from ordinary or medicinal leeches. Leech was also the name given to early doctors so a physician may have owned the land.

Dr Henry Proctor reporting bleeding a patient who was exhausted and semiconscious after a fight. Perhaps not unnaturally it was ineffective, and the patient subsequently died.[11]

Leeches still have a specific role in modern medicine due to their anticoagulation (blood thinning) properties.

Hermeticists.

An offshoot of the 'conventional' medicine of the day in the 16th century was the Hermeticists. Their best-known exponent was the renowned Welsh poet and doctor Henry Vaughan.

Hermeticists believed that all disease was caused by aspects of philosophy, particularly astrological ones. While their practice was seen as an obscure form of religion with bizarre beliefs, they claimed success in curing diseases conventional doctors could not.

Vaughan's treatise on the right way to preserve and restore health was his most important medical work. It was a translation of the work of Henry Nollius. Amongst other things this laid down good practice for eating and drinking, the importance of fresh air and leading a righteous life.

Henry lived just 20 miles from Hay near Talybont on Usk, and is buried at St Bride's Church, Llansantffraed. The extent of his medical practice, and whether his teachings influenced anyone in the Hay area is unknown.

'New' treatments.

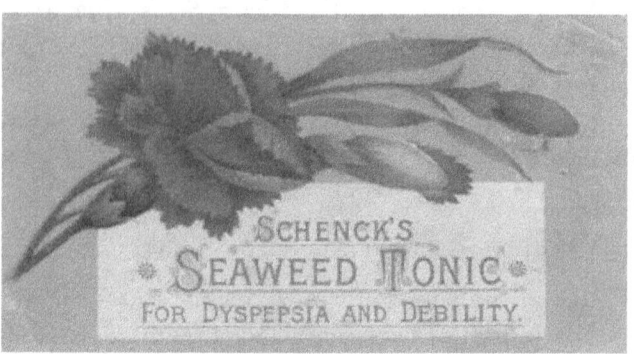

While rural Hay may have been far from the leading centres of medicine improved medical practice did gradually permeate through to the countryside.

Places like Chester, Ludlow and Bristol acted as quasi capitals for the Welsh borderlands. Medical innovations started to percolate through to them from London, Edinburgh, and even Cardiff. From there they passed to towns such as Hereford and Leominster, which are not far from Hay.

In addition the spread was aided by prominent citizens such as Sir Thomas Aubrey of Llantrithyd who had medicines sent direct from London.[12]

From the early 1800's a number of preparations started to appear to supplement the traditional remedies.

Local and national papers carried advertisements for patent medicines. Typically these might be prepared by London surgeons but were made available nationally in towns like Hereford, where it was sold from the offices of the Hereford Times.[13]

Schenck's Pulmonic Syrup,

The best and most positive cure for Consumption, Coughs, Sore Throat, Hoarseness, Whooping Cough, and all other diseases of the throat, lungs and respiratory organs.

Schenck's Seaweed Tonic,

For Dyspepsia and Debility. This Tonic mixes with the gastric juices, aids digestion, and creates a healthy appetite.

Schenck's Mandrake Pills,

For all diseases of the Liver and Stomach. These pills contain no calomel, and are exclusively vegetable. They act directly upon the liver, and are valuable in all cases of Sick headache, Indigestion, and all other bilious disorders. See Schenck's Almanac, which can be had gratis of all druggists.

All of Dr. Schenck's Medicines are for sale by

J. Sibbald, M. D.,
NORTH WALES, PA.

- Congreave's Balsamic Elixir for Coughs, Shortness of Breath, Asthma, and Consumption.
- Abernethy's Pile Ointment.
- Dr Flemming's Quinine and Camphor Pills to counteract febrile action and treat all cases of Indigestion, Headache, Heartburn, Loss of appetite,…..Flatulence, Shortness of Breath, ….Spasms…etc. Dr Reece who had a practice in Hay at the time provided a reference.
- Frank's Specific Solution of Copaiba for the cure of all Urethral discharges, Gleets (discharge from gonorrhoea), spasmodic strictures, irritation of the kidneys, bladder, urethra and prostate gland. This was referenced by three eminent London surgeons.
- Yolande Solution was promoted for the curing of gonorrhoea, and all associated conditions of the urinary tract, similar to the Solution of Copaiba. It claimed that after treatment Mrs Anne Spillane passed a urinary stone three and a half inches long, four and a quarter in circumference and weighing one and a half ounces.[14]
- Frank's Sarsine Paste, a Compound of Sarsaparilla, was advertised 'to treat Rheumatic Gout and all Neuralgic Affections, including impairment from the use/abuse of Mercury' (used to treat venereal disease).
- Rowland's produced Macassar Oil to nourish hair and prevent greying, as well as Kalydor to 'eradicate Eruptions, Tan, Pimples, Freckles, Redness and Spots'.

- Dr Locock's Pulmonic Wafers cured colds, asthma and consumption.
- A similar product Ford's Pectoral Balsam of Horehound also cured influenza.
- Snooks Aperient Family Pills for bilious and liver complaints, as well as indigestion, giddiness, loss of appetite, flatulence, spasms and costiveness (constipation).[15]

In 1838 a surgeon dentist from Hay, Mr Bayes, advertised Bayes invaluable Disinfecting Solution, suitable for the delicate of both sexes, for the prevention and treatment of 'A Certain Complaint' i.e. venereal disease.[16]

The famous diarist Rev. Francis Kilvert was ill on a number of occasions and recorded details of his treatment. On the 5 March 1878 Lady Cornewall gave him a bottle of Syrup of Hypophosphate of Lime when he complained of congested lungs. Today we know that this acts as a stimulant and increases the production of saliva.

Later that year on the 7 December he had a sore throat. Mr Giles suggested painting the back of his throat with tannin and glycerine, a common treatment at the time.

Arsenic.

For centuries arsenic has occupied a schizophrenic role in the health of the population. Just 0.145 grams, two grains (there are 437 grains in one ounce), or one eighth of a teaspoon of this white powder are enough to kill an adult person. The symptoms can be difficult to detect as they tend to mimic food poisoning, and as a consequence have featured in a number of high-profile criminal trials.

Despite this up until Victorian times it was widely available to buy by the general public as it was widely used as a rat poison and weedkiller. It was also an essential component in the Victorian doctor's arsenal of treatments.

Fowlers solution of 1% potassium arsenite was discovered in 1786 and became very popular. Fowlers was the medicine of choice to treat malaria, asthma, diphtheria, gastric ulcers and tuberculosis. Arsenic also had a role in the care of those with mental disease.

An arsenic based medicine Salvarsan was used to treat syphilis until the advent of penicillin. As late as the 1960's an arsenic based medicine was still being used to treat skin disease, apparently with positive results. Arsenic mixtures were second only to opium in the doctor's arsenal of treatments.[17]

The Arsenic Act of 1851 made it illegal to sell this white powder unless it was artificially coloured. The addition of charcoal or other dye meant is could not be ingested accidentally or administered unknowingly as a poison. Despite this, accidents did happen and people died when it was mistakenly used to replace glucose in sweets or beer, or as a whitening agent in bread.

Arsenic is only known to have caused one death in Hay. This was in the notorious case of the Hay Solicitor Herbert Rowse Armstrong, convicted (controversially) of poisoning his wife, Katherine.

Armstrong was convicted despite Katherine having been given an arsenic medicine when she was an inmate of Barnwood Lunatic Asylum shortly before her death.[18] Katherine was also a believer in homeopathy for a number of symptoms currently believed to indicate parathyroid disease. Her medicine of choice was a dilute arsenic solution arsenicum album, a solution still in the homeopath's arsenal of treatments.

Hay General Practitioner Dr Tom Hincks was closely involved in the trial.

Notes.

[1] Withey, Alun, Unhealthy Neglect? The Medicine and Medical Historiography of early Modern Wales, in *Social History of Medicine*, vol. 21, no. 1, Oxford University Press (2008) 163-74.

[2] Sarkey, J., *The Medicine Tree. Traditional Healing in Wales from pre-history to the present*, Llanerch Press (Lampeter, 2009).

[3] Jessica Furner-Pardoe, Blessing O. Anonye, Ricky Cain, et all. Anti-biofilm efficacy of a medieval treatment for bacterial infection requires the combination of multiple ingredients, *Scientific Reports* volume 10, Article number: 12687 (2020). https://doi.org/10.1038/s41598-020-69273-8.

[4] Letter by Miss Sarah A. Pape, F.R.C.S. Ed. (Plast.) in the *Daily Mail* (2017).

[5] Gies, J. and F. *Life in the Medieval Castle*, HarperCollins Publishers Ltd (2015).

[6] Palmer, Roy, *Folklore of Radnorshire,* Logaston Press (2001).

[7] Leather, E. M., *The Folk-Lore of Herefordshire*. Jakeman and Carver (1912). Reprinted by Lapridge Publications (1991).

[8] Recipe from Berrington Hall, Leominster.

[9] Stapleton, Edward J., *An Evacuee in the Hay and other stories.* (2012).

[10] *Hereford Journal* (14April 1852).

[11] *Hereford Journal* (2 April 1834).

[12] Bowen, J., ed., *Family and Society in Early Stuart Glamorganshire: The Household Accounts of Sir Thomas Aubrey of Llantrithyd, c.1565-1641*, South Wales Record Society (Cardiff, 2006).

[13] *Hereford Times* (29 September 1838).

[14] *Hereford Times* (9 February 1839).

[15] *Hereford Times* (25 November 1848).

[16] *Hereford Times.* (6 October 1838).

[17] Willcox, Phillip, *The Detective-Physician - The Life and Work of Sir Phillip Wilcox 1870 - 1941.* Heinemann Medical Books (1970).

[18] Beales, Martin, *The Hay Poisoner.* CPI Group Ltd. (1975).

Chapter 2 – Disease

In medieval times the spectre of disease constantly hovered over everybody. The population was prone to a number of maladies that are almost unknown today but, in those days, would spread through families like wildfire.

Ergotism.

Rye was the grain of the poor man in the Middle Ages as wheat was too expensive. This was particularly so in Wales where the only good wheat growing area was in the north around Anglesey.

Unfortunately when rye becomes damp it is prone to a fungus which forms dark purple or black bodies in the heads of grain. These ergots are responsible for a disease that causes symptoms of seizures, headaches and gastrointestinal disorders. A second form of it causes loss of skin sensation, oedema (swelling), gangrenous peeling of the skin, and ultimately tissue death.

At the time this disease was known as St Anthony's Fire or Holy Fire. While it almost certainly occurred locally there is no record of any outbreak in Hay.

Leprosy or Hanson's disease (*mycobacterium leprae*).

Leprosy is a bacterial disease causing damage to nerves, the respiratory system, skin and eyes. It damages nerve endings, meaning sufferers cease to feel pain. This results in damage to the extremities from unnoticed injury or infection. Over time these would become gangrenous and fall off, and weeping ulcers would develop in the face, mouth, throat and eyes.

Despite its low rate of infection it was a greatly feared disease in medieval times. It was not particularly uncommon as anyone with skin disease like eczema or psoriasis would be included. Sufferers were shunned by society. They were forced to wear a cloak and ring a bell wherever you went.

Not only did it have devastating physical effects. It had a reputation as a corrupting influence as it was generally believed to be the result of a licentious, immoral life and mortal sin. Because of this stigma leprosy was renamed Hanson's disease in the 20th century.

Fortunately Hay seems to have been relatively virtuous as only two cases can be traced to the town, one in the days of King Stephen and one later in 1208 during the reign of King John. By 1400 the prevalence of the disease had generally rapidly declined.

Plague (*yersinia pestis*).

There are records of plagues in Wales from the sixth century, but these outbreaks are generally referred to as the Yellow Plague. Not a great deal is known about them as details are lost in the mists of time.[1]

To modern historians plague means the bubonic version, the Great Plague, later known as the Black Death. It is known to have caused the deadliest pandemic in history although fortunately it is now rare and easily treated with antibiotics. For centuries it devastated Europe and Asia killing millions of people. It was known as The Great Pestilence or The Great Mortality, and at the time no one knew what caused it.

To many it was God's judgement. A French Doctor Guy de Chauliac suggested in 1345 that it was caused by the juxtaposition of three great planets, Saturn, Jupiter and Mars. Such an event was believed to be a sign of wonderful, terrible or violent things to come. His advice 'Go quickly, go far, and return slowly'

Suggestions on how it spread included looking at a victim, breathing 'bad air' or drinking contaminated water. Every nation tended to blame another.

For over two centuries it has been accepted that the source of the plague bacterium was a bite from the black rat flea, which was also responsible for its spread. This view is being revised and current thinking is that it was spread by human fleas and body lice.

However it spread the insanitary conditions in towns exacerbated the spread, and conditions in the countryside were little better. The Welsh population on the hills suffered as much as the English in the lower lying valleys and coastal plains.

Plague first reached South Wales during the winter of 1348-49. This was around the same time it affected the rest of the country. Many areas were very badly affected but Hay, along with Brecon and Huntington, appear to have got off relatively lightly.

They were off the main communication routes and relatively isolated.

Another visitation in 1361 only seems to have affected limited areas of West Wales. It was the outbreak in 1369, known as the Second Pestilence, that badly affected Southeast Wales including Hay.

The plague returned periodically for several centuries but was often localised. Communities tried to isolate themselves in the countryside at its onset. This was not always successful and only three inhabitants of Presteigne were left after a visitation in the 1630's.

Amongst numerous preventative ideas suggested were:

- Throwing sweet smelling herbs on the fire.
- Sitting in a sewer where the bad air drove off the less bad air of the plague.
- Killing all the cats and dogs in town.
- Self-flagellation.

Faith was often put in amulets, either worn on the arm or around the neck. Textual amulets were particularly popular, and often worn over the heart. More spectacular cures were equally unsuccessful.

- Drinking 10-year-old treacle as a medicine.
- Swallowing crushed emeralds or arsenic powder.
- Bloodletting.
- Having a live chicken strapped to the pustules.[2]

While all these fanciful theories have captured the public imagination, other simpler actions were taken and were effective to an extent. Infected persons were locked in their houses to quarantine them. The clothes trade was stopped. People walked in the middle of the road to avoid others, and reputedly coins in shops were dropped in vinegar to disinfect them. These methods proved to be effective. Could it be this experience is why the Sage Committee adopted a similar approach to Coved 19?[3]

There was also a medieval disinfecting protocol using brimstone, saltpetre and amber. Modern research has demonstrated that this system of fumigation, followed by limewashing, is very effective at killing viruses similar to Covid.

We do not have any accurate figures for the mortality rate of the plague for the whole of the United Kingdom. In individual areas mortality rates in excess of 50% are common. Moneyed classes complained of a shortage of servants, craftsmen and labourers,[4] but it is the reduction in rental income from tenant farmers that has been taken as the best guide to the mortality.

The general consensus now is that the population of Britain of around six million was reduced by at least a third and possibly as much as two thirds. The effect of these changes in agriculture was the decline of the traditional manor farm.

With the shortage of labour big estates could no longer function in their traditional way and land was rented out. Corn growing was discontinued. Sheep farming became more extensive, particularly so in the Bohun estates which included Hay.

This led to a rise in independent farming which in turn made the population as a whole wealthier. As a consequence people were able to increase their standard of living, and so general health improved.

There were other health consequences of the plague. It affected the conduct of war. The reduced population made it more difficult to recruit sufficient men for an army. Owain Glyndwr lost many men to the plague in 1403 at the siege of Caernarvon. This affected his subsequent campaigning.

The fact he never attacked Hay despite being in Brecknockshire may be due to this. Not only was the town spared from being sacked but it also avoided a plague visitation brought by the visiting soldiers.

Sweating Sickness (*sudor Anglicus* - the English sweat).

This uniquely English disease occurred six times in the late 15th and 16th centuries. It was a form of influenza and victims usually died within hours. Initially victims felt cold and developed a headache with aching limbs. This was followed minutes to hours later by heavy sweating. Anyone who lasted 24 hours usually survived.

Unlike influenza it normally occurred in the summer and affected young fit people, hence its rapid spread in large bodies of men such as armies.

It only occurred on the continent twice. Firstly it was among the English soldiers at Calais in 1502. The second occasion was in the fourth visitation of 1528-9. It swept across north-eastern Europe from the Netherlands to Switzerland, on through Poland and into Russia. Then it died out.

Hay was fortunate. After the Norman conquest of Wales it remained off the beaten track. No invading armies passing through. This may be why no cases have been recorded in the town. Its most prominent victim was probably Henry VII's son Arthur Prince of Wales when he was at Ludlow in 1502.

In later centuries diseases such as these became rare. Unfortunately they were replaced by others such as typhoid fever, tuberculosis, cholera and smallpox, to all of which country folk had little immunity.

Typhoid Fever *(salmonella enterica subsp)*.
Typhoid fever causes a high temperature before gangrene affects fingers and toes. It is caused by a salmonella bug from ingestion of faecal material due to poor sanitation and hygiene.

In the past outbreaks were associated with large companies of men, such as a passing army, and was often in addition to an outbreak of syphilis. Typhoid has its origin in poor sanitation, and before the advent of a general improvement in water supplies it occurred in rural areas just as much as in cities.

In Hay the medical officer reported there were three outbreaks in 1856 with one fatality. Following another case in 1879 the medical officer Dr Clouston ordered an immediate inspection of the drains.

In 1905 there was one case at Mr Howards, the blacksmith on Bell Bank.

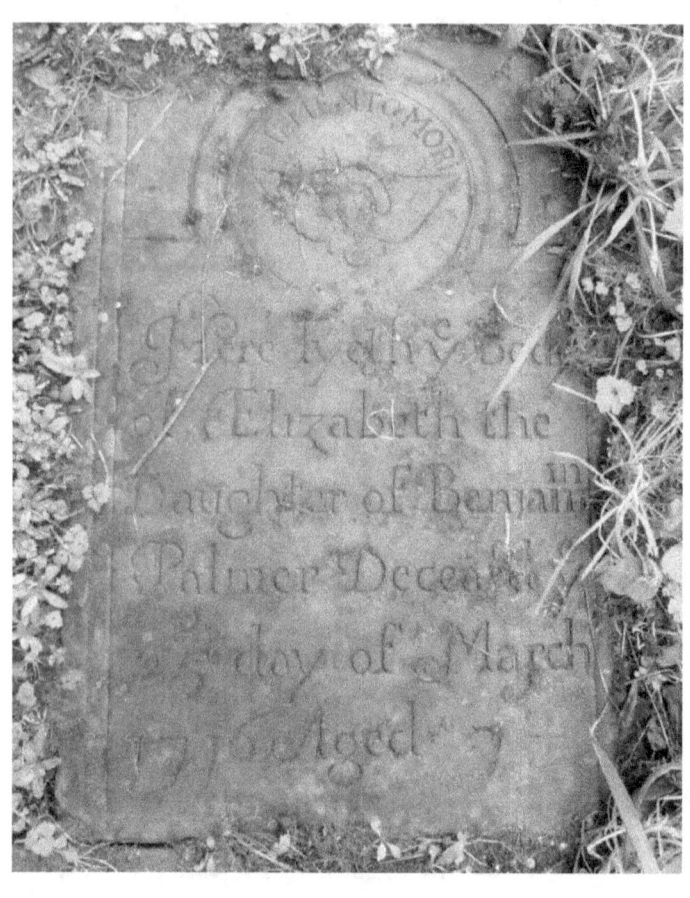

A grave marker for a 7-year-old child in Hay churchyard.

Tuberculosis or TB *(mycobacterium tuberculosis)*.

As leprosy declined so TB, or consumption as it was known, was on the increase. This respiratory disease was common throughout the country for centuries. Around 90% of victims did not show any symptoms but of the 10% who did around half died. It was the commonest cause of death at the beginning of the 19th century.

The majority of people were exposed to it although as they grew older they developed a basic immunity. Despite this it took a steady toll of relatively young individuals. It was not unknown for whole families living in the same house to infect one another and die.

Spare a thought for Thomas Cartwright of Hay. He buried two children in infancy, Ann in 1814 and George in 1819. This at a time when child mortality rates were anything up to 40%. In 1827 he buried his son John aged 20 years and then in 1829 William aged 19 years. Finally in 1830 he buried his last son George and his wife Ann aged 48 years.

Although we will never know the causes of death, given the three-year timescale of his elder sons and wife, TB in the family must be the prime suspect.

We do know of deaths that were certainly due to it. On the 9 June 1872 Rev. Francis Kilvert recorded in his diary that Mrs Prosser 'a young pretty woman' at the Swan Hotel was dying of consumption. It was assumed that she caught it from her sister Mrs Hope of the Rose and Crown in Broad Street.

It also seems to have been the cause of death recorded on two grave markers in St Mary's churchyard, Hay.

An inscription on the grave of Mary, wife of William Price, who died 1 December 1765 aged 27 years reads:

With wasting pain, Death found me long oppressed,
Pitied my sighs and kindly brought me rest.

George Lewis junior, who died 29 June 1807 aged 23 years, has the simple inscription:

Pale consumption gave the fatal blow.

In his 1913 annual report Dr Tom Hincks reported that he was called to visit two TB cases in the district.

Concern about the prevalence of this disease led to the formation of the King Edward VII Welsh National Memorial Association, with the aim to treat and eradicate tuberculosis in Wales. In 1912 thirteen separate districts in Wales were designated, each with their own dedicated physician, and with a central base in Cardiff.

In a survey the association found that 70% of adults and 43% of children in Wales showed signs of the infection, and 30% of adult and 21% of child contacts actually had the disease.

After the First World War the Public Health (Tuberculosis) Act 1921 required local authorities to treat and prevent the disease. In Wales the King Ed. VII Association took on this task and it set up hospitals specifically to treat TB cases. The South Wales Sanitorium at Bronllys, eight miles from Hay, with its 304 beds was the largest in the United Kingdom. It was opened by King George V and Queen Mary in 1920.[5]

Cholera.

> **NOTICE.**
>
> **PREVENTIVES OF CHOLERA!**
>
> Published by order of the Sanatory Committee, under the sanction of the Medical Counsel.
>
> **BE TEMPERATE IN EATING & DRINKING!**
> *Avoid Raw Vegetables and Unripe Fruit !*
> Abstain from **COLD WATER**, when heated, and above all from *Ardent Spirits*, and if habit have rendered them indispensable, take much less than usual.

Cholera did not arrive in the United Kingdom, from India, until around 1819 but it thrived in the heavy urbanised areas that grew up in the 19th century.

Between 1830 and 1860 40,000 Londoners died from the disease, but it had already been rife throughout South Wales between 1820 and 1840. In a short article headed 'Cholera' in the Hereford Times October 1832 a general decline in the pestilence was reported, with the exception of Worcester, Bristol and Merthyr Tydfil. The newspaper report went on to urge readers, for the sake of their health and avoiding cholera, to avoid wet feet under any circumstances.[6]

There was a particularly bad outbreak in South Wales in 1849, after which a Day of Humiliation was appointed by the Bishop of St David's. The Hereford Times reported:

.... a full sense of the solemnity of the occasion.
All business was suspended and inns and beer houses closed till after the service.
The exemption from cholera which hitherto has mercifully been granted to this parish and neighbourhood tended to redouble their zeal and devotion.[7]

The insanitary conditions and polluted water supplies in the industrial valleys were known to be responsible for outbreaks. Even before the actual cause of cholera had been discovered legislation was introduced. The 1846 and 1848 Nuisances Removal and Diseases Prevention Act required local boards to cover cesspits and foul drains to remove pools of stagnant water.

In Hay William Acton the High Bailiff issued a proclamation about taking precautions. A committee under George Jones was tasked to 'patrol the town and report nuisances' suggesting their removal. Typical precautions included the removal of pigsties, refuse heaps and open drains. Castle Street was noted to be the worst due to the number of pigs rooting in the refuse left outside doors.

In practice Hay was fortunate. It was a rural area with a relatively low density of population. It also had a clean water supply from the local wellsprings, and good drainage of polluted water into the Wye. As a consequence it was relatively spared the disease.

In contrast the heavily polluted River Hondu in Brecon caused a bad outbreak in 1849. At the time Dr Thomas Prestwood Lucas of Brecon undertook pioneering work to trace the underlying cause of the disease. Unfortunately, despite getting close, he was unsuccessful.

It was not until the early 1850's that Dr John Snow demonstrated cholera was caused by polluted water supplies. After this preventative measures were put in place nationally and fortunately this caused a rapid decline in cases.

Despite this Hay still had problems. In 1853[8] a concerned citizen wrote to the Hereford Times deploring the state of the town, a situation again reported in the newspaper in 1865.[9]

A lack of understanding of basic hygiene and germs led people to believe that contagious diseases were caught from bad smells or 'miasmas' as they were called. It was thought that cholera was spread this way from dead bodies.

As a consequence Local Boards of Health stipulated the time in which victims were to be buried. Ann Hopkins of Merthyr was fined £2 or 14 days imprisonment for refusing to bury her husband within this time.

Another device to prevent exposure to miasmas was the building of Dead Houses. Loved ones would lay there before burial, rather than in their homes or the local church. One of these rare buildings was constructed a few miles from Hay at Boughrood. It is not known if anyone from Hay used the facility.

Smallpox (*variola virus*).

Smallpox was the dominant cause of mortality in Europe in the 16th century, although in rural areas it was not generally a major problem as quarantine could be easily arranged.

Occasional cases of smallpox occurred in Hay, such as in October 1752 when the local curate had to bury his wife and daughter due to the disease.

> TALGARTH.—Births 18; deaths 20 Whooping-cough is prevalent, and has been fatal in two cases.
> HAY.—Births 34; deaths 30. Small-pox has prevailed, but has not been very fatal. There were five deaths from small-pox. Low typhoid fever has also prevailed, and caused four deaths.

A newspaper extract showing that in 1859 smallpox was prevalent in Hay.

This 1859 report stated that it was not as bad as previous outbreaks as it 'has not been very fatal' with only five deaths.[10] The incidence of typhoid fever was also thought to be low as it only caused four deaths.

Six years later in 1865 smallpox was more prevalent and lingered in the area for a number of weeks. This time there were two fatalities.

On the 17/18 May 1893 many visitors stayed away from the Spring Fair in Hay because one person in the town was infected. Fortunately the patient recovered and, due to the precautions taken, there were no other cases.

At the Board of Guardians meeting 1896 the issue of disinfecting the clothing of those who had smallpox arose. The town had installed a 'Disinfecting Apparatus' at the workhouse for the clothing of inmates. The question arose whether private persons could have access to it as it was paid for by public money. After discussion the board decided that it was open to the suggestion.

A committee was set up to examine and make recommendations on two issues. Firstly how to transport the clothing safely to the disinfecting room without infecting others, and then how to defray any additional expenses such as the coal involved.[11]

While the local population might take precautions, the itinerant vagrants who could spread the disease were a constant cause for concern. This was not unfounded as it was due to visitations of vagrants that there were cases in 1902 and 1903. On each occasion isolation was arranged, in the first case by placing the victim in a tent in the ruins of Cardigan Hall, a house on the hill above the graveyard. (See Isolation Hospital later).

Hay had a predominantly sheep rather than dairy based economy so it is unlikely much immunity from smallpox would have been acquired following cowpox infection. However once the link between cowpox and smallpox was established, and the value of vaccination established by Edward Jenner, the prevalence of smallpox declined nationally.

Following a sustained international vaccination programme the last recorded case of smallpox was in 1978. Ironically that was in the United Kingdom. It was declared globally eradicated in 1980.

With increased knowledge, and suitable preventative measures, the prevalence of typhoid fever, cholera and smallpox declined rapidly. Unfortunately there were a number of other endemic infectious diseases to take their place.

Diphtheria (*Corynebacterium diphtheriae*).

Diphtheria was a relatively common but serious bacterial infection until after the Second World War. It creates a toxin which affects the nose and throat, causing breathing difficulty, heart failure and paralysis. It can be fatal. In 1878 Queen Victoria's daughter Princess Alice and Princess Marie of Hesse died of it.

In a sketch of medical practice in Radnorshire in the 1890's mention is made of a doctor's visit to an isolated farmhouse to attend one boy who had breathing difficulty. After he succumbed to the disease one by one his siblings died of the same cause, six in all.[12]

In 1897 there were two cases in Oak Row, Hay, one of which was fatal. We now know it is spread by direct transmission, but these cases were blamed on the Loggin Brook. Then it was an open watercourse at the side of Brecon Road and used as the main town drain. Further cases in Hay occurred periodically including 1903, 1929, 1930 and 1934.

The author had a 14-year-old aunt who died of the disease in the epidemic that swept Europe in 1942-43.

Whooping Cough (*pertussis*).

Whooping cough is a horrible disease of relatively recent origin, having first been recorded in Paris in 1414. Since then it has rapidly spread and become endemic throughout Europe. Hay suffered as much as elsewhere, although it appears to have avoided the whooping cough outbreak that was prevalent in

Talgarth and which resulted in two deaths in 1859.[13] It was a recurrent problem and led to the closure of the schools in Hay on a number of occasions such as 3 June to 31 August 1901.

Scarlet Fever (*Streptococcus pyogenes*).

Scarlet fever is a streptococcal infection and was responsible for between 10,000 and 34,000 deaths a year in the United Kingdom between 1853-80. There were outbreaks approximately every 4 years. It was a leading cause of death in infants in the early 20th century.

The minutes of the Local Board in 1859 reported that low levels of scarlet fever that year had resulted in only four deaths.[14] This was not always the case and in other years numbers were much higher.

The Rev. Francis Kilvert went to visit a sick child Meredith in November 1870. While he was there Meredith's mother had told him that Meredith's sister Catherine had scarlet fever. This was diagnosed after she had a fever and sore throat, and the skin on her hands started to peel. It seems this was treated with general indifference. No precautions against the spreading of infection or the use of any sort of disinfection were taken.

It was after an epidemic in 1879-80 that Benjamin Whishlade, a builder from Kington, was appointed to conduct an enquiry in Hay. We do not have the report but we know that as the disease was highly contagious it concentrated on cleanliness and the prevailing insanitary conditions. He made a number of recommendations.

- Isolate victims.
- All cottages to be whitewashed with limewash and carbolic acid. Traps and sewers to be disinfected.
- Notices to be distributed emphasising isolation and enforcing the use of disinfectants.
- Straw bedding to be destroyed.
- Quick burial of victims.
- Take action against those exposing themselves to others while suffering from the infection.
- Where death occurred, houses to be limewashed again.

At the same time Dr Shepherd was asked to analyse the water of the Black Lion and the Town Wells. The piped water from the reservoirs on Hay Common was also felt to be in an impure state. The clerk was asked to write to the owners to analyse the water and confirm it was satisfactory. All this led Dr Shepherd to request an increase in remuneration from £5 to £20 per annum.

Whishlade's report was so critical that the Local Board met six times over the following twelve days to rectify the concerns highlighted. Meanwhile the Inspector of Nuisances was sacked. Whishlade's recommendations were endorsed when shortly afterwards both the Lancet and British Medical Journal (B.M.J.) published guidance papers. These emphasised isolation of victims, and the need to avoid overcrowding and unsanitary conditions.

Despite this outbreaks were still frequent. They were reported in 1881, 1893, and throughout 1894.

There were further cases and multiple school closures in 1895 and 1896. In 1902 outbreaks occurred in Heol y Dwr and Newport Street.

One patient ended up being isolated in a cottage in Oxford Road, but for the outbreaks in 1912 and 1914 the newly opened isolation hospital was used.

Measles (*Morbillivirus*).

Measles is one of the most highly infectious diseases, and it can lead to potentially serious complications such as brain and eye damage.

Records of it are scant in Hay but in 1893 a resident of Gypsy Castle was put into temporary isolation due to it. The school was shut in January 1896 for two months due to outbreaks in the town.

Infection (wound fever).

While not a disease in itself infection was a very real hazard before the age of antibiotics. Its prevalence led it to be known as wound fever and it undoubtedly claimed numerous lives. Any wound, however small, could become infected in one of two ways.

- Tetanus (*Clostridium tetani*).
  If a wound came in contact with the soil or manure tetanus could result. The symptoms were muscle stiffness leading to spasms and an inability to move the jaw – hence the name lockjaw. Swallowing became increasingly difficult, and muscle spasm meant breathing became laboured and eventually the patient suffocated.

- Septicaemia.
  If tetanus was avoided it was taken as normal for any cut or abrasion to acquire at least a mild infection. If this became severe, and developed into sepsis where the whole body's immune system reacted, death was the result.

Living conditions started to improve in Victorian times. As a result complications from these diseases started to reduce due to improvements in sanitation, housing and public health rather than medical advances.

Equally important was improved nutrition which made people generally healthier and better able to combat disease. This was difficult if you were poor but as the nation became wealthier a number of charities were founded to help this section of society.

Almshouses.

From the Middle Ages charitable 'hospitals' had been set up to help the poorest sections of society, providing sheltered accommodation and support. Gradually they evolved into almshouses, and most came into existence before the era of the workhouse.

They were not care homes and residents had to be fit enough to look after themselves, but too poor to be able to afford their own accommodation. Their main advantage was the freedom residents were allowed compared to that they would get in the workhouse.

Two sets of almshouses were erected in Hay.
- The Gwynne Almshouses.

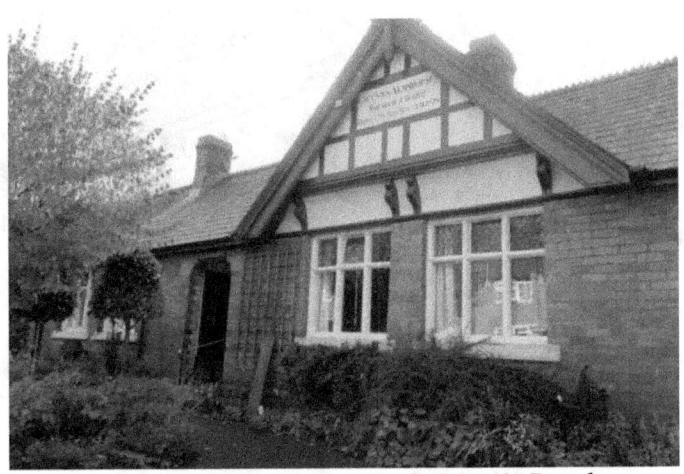

The Gwynne Almshouses in St Mary's Road

Elizabeth Gwynne endowed 'a habitation for six of the most poor, weak, and indigent people of' Hay in her will dated 31 January 1699. Originally this was built in Chain Alley, off Wyeford Road. She also left land, the rent from which provided money for their support. Unfortunately the original terms made no provision for maintenance of the property and it fell into disrepair. By the 1850's it had become uninhabitable. A new building to replace it was built in St Mary's Road, near the church, in 1878.

- The Harley Almshouses.

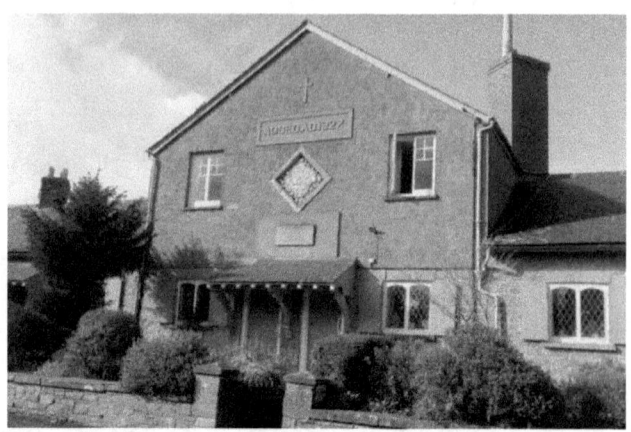

The Harley Almshouses in Brecon Road.

Frances Harley of Trebarried endowed six houses in Church Street in memory of her mother in 1832, and a further set of twelve in Brecon Road in memory of her sister four years later.[15]

> WORTHY OF IMITATION.—Six Alms Houses for as many indigent poor women have been lately erected in the Hay, by a most benevolent lady, and the interior of them are now nearly completed, and fit for the reception of inmates. They have a particularly neat appearance, are substantially built of stone with slated roof, and each house comprises a sitting and a sleeping room sufficiently spacious, with excellent fire-places and closets, and behind is a garden. On the front of the buildings are the family arms neatly carved on stone, and below the following inscription—
>
> These Alms Houses were erected
> And Endowed by Frances Harley
> To the Memory of her Mother,
> The HONOURABLE MRS. HARLEY
> Of Trebarried—For the reception
> Of 6 Poor Indigent Women,
> A.D. MDCCCXXXII.

In 1927 an upper floor was added to the Brecon Road property as a matrons flat, and all were updated in 1974 when individual residential units were enlarged and reduced to four and eight respectively.

Residents of almshouses were almost invariably widows. Whether they were exceptional or not we do not know, but being poor does not appear to have been a reason for a short lifespan.

In 1825 the Cambrian newspaper reported that in one set of almshouses in Hay there lived Ann Watkins aged 105 years and her daughter aged 75 years.

The paper commented that:

'a fact proving the salubrity of the air in that part of the country, which is remarkable for the longevity of its inhabitants'.[16]

Earlier it had reported that the combined ages of four widows in the almshouses was 329 years.[17]

Friendly Societies.

During the 19th century a number of friendly societies were established in Hay. In addition to their philanthropic work they ran contributory insurance schemes to support the poor in times of sickness, or the costs of a funeral. The Rev. Frances Kilvert refers to attending some of their fetes.

The Amicable Friendly Society (male) was based in the Rose and Crown Inn Broad Street. Established on 24 November 1835[18] the Amicable was said to have the most influential members. Each year it hosted a parade, led by their band, to St Mary's church.

Dr Henry Proctor was the appointed medical officer in 1850. Other similar societies were based at the Black Lion and the Union at the George.

Societies often held parades after which a banquet would be held at which the toasting could go on until 4 am. There were claims that these were little more than drinking clubs but despite this reputation clergy were members. The tomb of the Rev. Richard Lloyd was erected in 1797 by a friendly society based at the Black Lion.

The Loyal Favourable Design Lodge of the Order of Oddfellows was established in Hay in 1838. On their first anniversary they held a church service 'accompanied by a large portion of the St John's Lodge Brecon' followed by 'a most excellent dinner'.[19]

In 1842 Dr Ebenezer Reece was their resident medical officer He was able to provide advice to support the orders aim, which hasn't changed to the present day - to 'visit the sick, relieve the distressed, bury the dead and educate the orphan'. There were branches at Hereford, Brilley, Eardisley, Pembridge, Dorstone, Glasbury, Talgarth, Kington and Radnor.

Another society the Ancient Order of Foresters, 'Court Perseverance' no. 4906, was established in 1866. They met in the Wheatsheaf Inn, Lion Street.[20] Within three years of being established it had 65 members. Again the order formed its own band.

The Foresters sponsored an Athletic Festival and Sports in 1903 at the football club. Entrants were said to include 'First-Class Athletes' from across the country and a handicapping system was promised to allow locals to compete on equal terms. The band of D

Company the 1st Volunteer Battalion South Wales Borderers under Capt. Dr Tom Hincks played during the afternoon.[21]

The order obviously only recruited fit members, or it was keen to ensure that its members maintained a good level of fitness. On the Festival Day they met at the Parish Hall at 9a.m., and proceeded to St Mary's church for a service. Then they paraded through town to The Moor on the Hardwicke Road before going up to Llydyadway in Cusop. These were the homes of prominent members. By this time it must have been late morning as they paraded to the football ground in Brecon Road, a total distance of around five miles altogether. Lunch was provided. Then they were able to enjoy the afternoon's entertainment.[22]

Hay also had a branch of the Order of Rechabites, a teetotal friendly society who operated an insurance and savings scheme. Branches were known as 'Tents' with a 'Junior Tent' for children.

In 1904 they met in 'the tent room' in Lion Street, presumably either the Drill Hall or the Parish Rooms. The Rechabites were supporters of the Hay Total Abstinence Society. That year the Abstinence Society met in the Salvation Army Barracks 'to celebrate a very successful year'.

Other philanthropic organisations were the Loyal Hay Lodge of Freemasons No 2382 and the brethren of the Welsh Border Lodge no. 905 of the Royal Ancient Order of Buffalos (R.A.O.B.).

It is interesting to note that the names of the members and officials of these various organisations were the same time and time again.

The presidents, chairs, etc. were often worthies such as the Rev. J.J. de Winton, Major E.F. Cockcroft, Major E.H. Cheese, Major W.H. Booth, Col. Garnons-Williams, or the Hon. R.C. Deveraux.

Members were major landholders or merchants such as H.R. Grant, J.M. Maddy, William Giles, W. Lillwall, C. Kedward, W. Pugh, F.B. Powell, T.J. Stokoe, and C.E. Tunnard-Moore. Such people were the monied middle class who combined their leisure interests with their social consciences.

Support by the Friendly Societies, combined with the introduction of a weekly pension of 25p from 1 January 1909 for all persons over 70 years, were major steps forward in improving the health of the poorest sections of the community. This was bolstered further by the provisions of the National Insurance Act of 1911.[23]

Finally in 1948 the National Insurance Scheme and the founding of the National Health Service secured a safety net for all those in need of medical care.

Interestingly the Foresters objected strongly to one specific provision in the Act. It stated that 'there was no place for friendly societies in the administration of the new scheme of insurance'.[24] Perhaps they could see that this did away with much of the philanthropic purpose for which friendly societies were originally established. Interest in most of them rapidly dwindled during the 1960's and 70's.

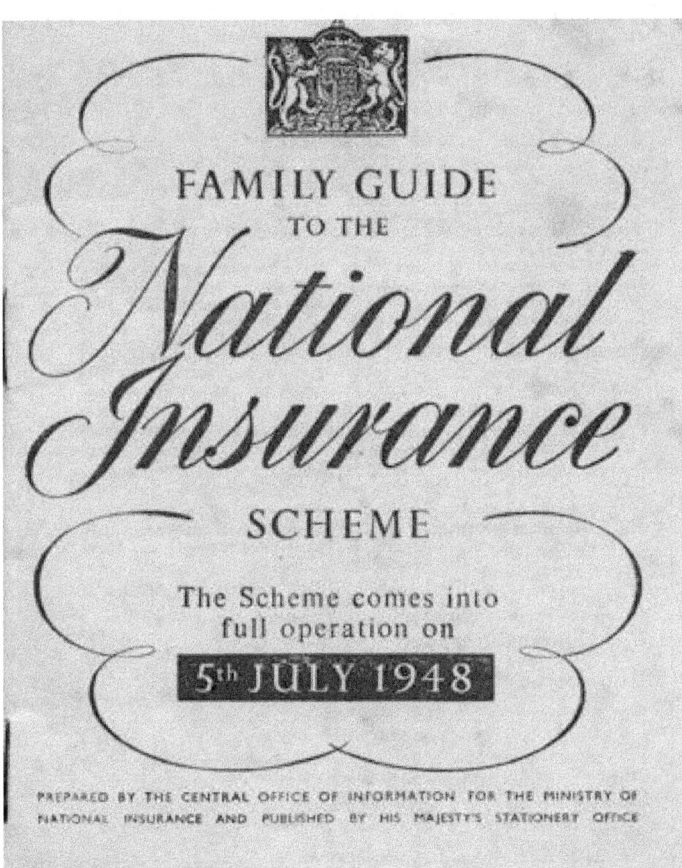

Notes.

[1] Cule, J., *Wales and Medicine,* J.D. Lewis and Sons Ltd. (Llandysul, 1975) 141.

[2] Deary, T. and Brown, M., *Horrible Histories Measly Middle Ages,* Scholastic (London, 1996).

[3] Alberge, Dalya, Virus measures echo Great Plague response, *Sunday Telegraph* (8 November 2020) 17.

[4] *Historia Roffensis* British Library.

[5] Cule, J., *Wales and Medicine,* J.D. Lewis and Sons Ltd. (Llandysul, 1975) 32.

[6] *Hereford Times* (6 October1832).

[7] *Hereford Times* (20 October 1849).

[8] *Hereford Times* (15 October 1853).

[9] *Hereford Times* (24 June 1865).

[10] *Welshman* (1st December 1859).

[11] *Brecon County Times* (17 April 1896).

[12] Anonymous, Medical Practice in Radnorshire, *Transactions of the Radnorshire Society* (1933) 27–35.

[13] *Welshman* (1 December 1859).

[14] *Welshman* (1 December 1859).

[15] *Monmouth Merlin* (13 October 1832).

[16] *Cambrian* (1 January 1825).

[17] *Cambrian* (25 May 1822).

[18] Parliamentary Papers, *The Accounts and Papers of the House of Commons vol. 51.* www.books.google.co.uk.

[19] *Hereford Journal* (3 July 1839).

[20] *Hay Parish Magazine* (1879, 80, 82, 85, 86, 88, 89)

[21] *Brecon County Times* (17 July 1903).

[22] *Brecon County Times* (29 July 1904).

[23] Hay Millennium Society, *Nobody has heard of Hay,* Logaston Press (Almerly, 2000).

[24] *Staffordshire Sentinel* (4 February 1946).

Chapter 3 – Emergency Medicine

Emergency Surgery.

In an age of good communications, and when all surgery is done in hospitals, it is difficult to appreciate just how different things were prior to the First World War.

For a rural doctor emergency surgery was all in a day's work. Patients would often postpone an operation as long as possible. Not only could it entail a long arduous journey to hospital, but also, and more importantly, there was the cost and the loss of income while recuperating. As a consequence, there were occasions when the delay gave rise to symptoms suddenly becoming worse. In addition, genuine unforeseen emergencies might be encountered.

In the absence of any means of quickly transferring a patient to hospital the doctor on the spot had to do what he could for his patients. Operations might have to be performed on the kitchen table, or even in the open air. This after a long journey over the hills, sometimes in pouring rain or driving snow, and possibly following multiple calls to isolated cottages.

A typical example was the Radnorshire country doctor who had to deal with a strangulated hernia in a small low-ceilinged farmhouse poorly lit by gas lamp.[1]

Accidents.

The countryside can be a dangerous place but it was even more so in the days of primitive machinery and a major dependence on horse-power. As a result there was always a constant stream of accidents, many of them fatal.

While we know of some of these, undoubtedly there would have been others that have gone unrecorded.

Following a landslip at the Kilkaning quarry, Maesllwsh estate, Glasbury, Evan James was almost covered in earth. He was released quickly by his colleagues but despite Dr Bogle's best efforts died of his injuries.[2]

In an incident on Hay bridge a horse and cart struck farmer William Price, knocking him off his horse. He was shaken and Mr Henry Proctor assessed a broken collar bone and two ribs. There did not appear to be any life-threatening injuries.

Mr Proctor saw Price over the next few days but unfortunately he died a fortnight later. At the post-mortem Mr Trumper found four broken ribs but said Price had died from badly congested lungs due to bronchitis. At 82 years of age the accident would have shaken him but it was not responsible for his death.[3]

Gamekeeper William Williams was shooting at Clifford when 'the gun he was using burst and inflicted serious wounds in his head and neck, rendering him for some time quite insensible'. Mr Reece was called and 'sewed up no less than seven wounds in the head of the sufferer'. The newspaper report continued 'He was afterwards conveyed to Hardwicke where we are glad to learn he is progressing most favourably.'[4]

The building trade has always provided a steady trade for the medical profession. In 1913 Dr Tom Hincks was called to The Moor on the Hardwick Road to attend Charles Thomas Evans who had fallen off the scaffolding. Unfortunately he had dislocated his neck and there was nothing medically that could be done for him. Perhaps at 67 years of age he was a little old to be running around scaffolding but before much in the way of social support retiring was often not an option.[5]

Any work involving felling trees is dangerous, even today. A young man named Parry, a relative of Mr W. Price of the Baskerville Arms Inn, was assisting a felling by pulling on a rope. The tree fell quicker than expected and he was hit, breaking his thigh. The newspaper reported that he was 'progressing favourably' under Dr Bogles care.[6]

Machinery.

Before the days of health and safety legislation, guards, etc., accidents involving machinery were a constant hazard.

A Mr Ambury had a serious accident when his leg was drawn between the rollers of a threshing machine and completely smashed. Mr Trumper and Mr Lloyde were called and amputated the limb the same night. Mr. Ambury recovered.[7]

At 2 pm on a Friday in August 1868 the railway station porter John Merrick was assisting in shunting goods trucks. This involved standing on the connecting bar between wagons, so he could climb up and apply the brake. His foot slipped and he fell backwards, hitting his head on the ground while the truck passed over his legs.

Merrick was carried to his nearby house where Dr Bogle attended him. After applying first aid and treatment for shock Dr Bogle recommended Merrick's immediate conveyance to the Infirmary in Hereford for amputation of both legs. A special train was prepared, and Merrick was placed on it attended by Dr Bogle.

For the first half of the journey his condition appeared stable but it deteriorated rapidly from there on and he was found to be dead on arrival.

The deceased was described as a very steady man who had been employed by the company for a number of years. Sadly he was a widower and left a family of four young children orphaned.[8]

Drowning.

With the River Wye so close to the town inevitable there were a steady stream of accidental drownings. The river looks very calm in the summer when the water level is low, but it can be deceptive. There is said to be a cold current into Steeple Pool, below the church, which can sweep the unsuspecting under and hold them down.

In 1850 William Price the 17yr old son of the landlord at the Rose and Crown Public House went down to swim after work. He got into difficulties and before help could arrive he drowned. Over 200 people attended his funeral and burial in St Mary's churchyard.

George Wood aged 17, son of a seedsman, drowned near Steeple Pool in July 1884 when he fell into a deep hole while bathing.[9]

Dr John Charles Taylor of Hay died when he fell from his horse crossing the Wye five miles upstream from Hay near Boughrood. He is buried in St Mary's graveyard Hay.

William Daniel Walkins, a 22-year-old draper, was returning home from Hay to Llanigon when the horse he was riding stumbled in a large brook. William was thrown off where the strong current swept him into the Wye.[10]

Alcohol.

Alcohol has always been a major contributor to the workload of the medical profession, and to fatalities. Charles Price a mason residing in the Gwynne Almshouses in Chain Alley, met his death by falling downstairs in a state of drunkenness in August 1866.[11]

In August 1869 there was an inquest into the death of Philip Pembridge a tailor in Hay who was 'addicted to drinking'. Mr Smith the surgeon attended when Pembridge was found dead one morning. The jury found that 'the deceased died from a fall down his cellar steps'.[12]

John Humphris of the Wine Vaults made a number of attempts on his life due to 'delirium tenens'. This is the confusion and hallucinations brought on by a rapid withdraw from alcohol. The first time it occurred he was unsuccessful at cutting his throat. Dr Bogle attended to him, leaving instructions that he should be supervised at all times.

Despite this Humphris made a second attempt. This also failed but he was more successful in injuring himself. Dr Lyde and Dr Bogle had to sew up his throat wound. Despite everyone's best efforts a few days later he died in his sleep following an excess intake of alcohol. He was only 33 years old.[13]

At an inquest on the butler from Clyro Court Dr Bogle stated that the 'brown blood' in the deceased's mouth indicated that he suffered from liver disease His death was most probably due to sclerosis of the liver causing the veins in his oesophagus (gullet) to rupture. Perhaps an occupational disease for a butler.

Animals.

Dr Bridgewater, with surgeons Mr Reese and Mr Lyde, attended William Lewis who was kicked in the stomach by a horse while out hunting with hounds at Wyeside. He died 24hours later.[14]

Dr Tom Hincks was called to Mr R.T. Griffiths when his horse bit him on the ear, necessitating a number of stitches.[15]

Children.

Paediatric care was less robust before vaccines and health screening. Disease followed by accidents caused most contact between doctors and children.

In December 1853 Dr Bogle was called to attend a child who had wet his pinafore. In the process of trying to dry it before an open fire 'it caught fire and enveloped him in a sheet of flame'. The boy was badly burnt and despite Dr Bogle's efforts he died the next day.[16]

The countryside is a wonderful playground but always potentially dangerous. Dr Hugh Powell was called to an accident where a five-year-old girl had fallen under the wheels of a threshing machine while it was being towed. Despite being aware of the child there was nothing the driver could have done to prevent it, and nothing the doctor could do for the child. She died shortly after he arrived.[17]

An eight-year-old boy Philip Williams, employed by wagoner Richard Evans, died when he was leading three horses pulling a cart. They ran away from him and when he ran to catch them he fell and the wheel went over his head. Mr Proctor was unable to do anything for Philip. Recording accidental death the jury deprecated the system of allowing boys of so tender an age to be entrusted with horses.[18]

Inevitably there were a number of instances where the doctors became involved in serious cases of ill harm to children.

Following evidence from sisters Jane and Clara Whitcombe the police found the body of a male child buried in a field. Mr Trumper and Mr Proctor were called to perform a post-mortem on the infant. Their conclusion was that the body was that of a full term healthy male infant. The lungs showed signs of inflation but the navel string 'had not been tied' and afterbirth was still attached. In their view the child had been born alive and appeared healthy with no signs of violence. It probably died from suffocation and want of attention after birth.

For some reason Dr Bogle was also called to examine the child post-mortem. He agreed with his colleagues that it died due to suffocation 'that may have been caused accidentally in many ways'. The doctors decided that there was nothing to indicate that the mother Jane Whitcombe 'had contributed to its death'. A week after the inquest the mother Jane together with her sister Clara were charged with concealing the birth and appeared at Clyro Petty Sessions. They were committed for trial at the Radnor Assizes.[19]

Dr Thomas Hincks was involved in a case of child cruelty. At Hay Petty Sessions a charge of ill treatment of a nine-year-old child, Thomas William Owens, was brought against Jane Hannah Owens and Mary Jane Owens of 2 Oxford Road.

Following a complaint Roderick Evans, the Brecon inspector for the N.S.P.C.C., called at 2 Oxford Road. On examining Thomas he found a number of injuries. When asked how they were caused the elder sister said, 'Polly did knock him about with her fist.' She admitted beating him with a stick because he slept out overnight. Asked why he did that Thomas said he was afraid to go back because they beat him.

Thomas was removed to the workhouse where Frank B. Powell the workhouse master said he was cowed, timid and depressed on admission but was now much brighter. Mr Powell found him truthful and a good boy in every respect.

Dr Hincks examination of Thomas found he had a black eye, with a slight cut and swollen bruise on the left side of his head. Both ears were blackened and there were marks of a stick or cane across his buttock. He said the injuries to the head were consistent with blows from the hand or fist and not a fall.

Thomas had lived with Mary Ann Clark of Almeley, for the previous eight years and looked upon her as his mother. She testified that he was always good and if he did anything wrong he always told her. The defendants were found guilty of ill treatment and fined £1 each. They were bound over for 12 months.[20]

Some forms of treatment were very primitive by modern standards. A simple operation like the removal of tonsils took on a different perspective when the child would have them sliced off without anaesthetic while sitting at the kitchen table.[21]

Childbirth.

Childbirth was a hazardous event until very recent times. The following examples were recorded in the surrounding area but undoubtedly Hay had its share of such tragedies.

- At New Radnor Priscilla Green aged 31 years died giving birth to her 20th child in 1731.
- A double tragedy occurred to one family at Disserth Radnorshire. In 1777 Sarah Hughlings aged 37 years died giving birth to a daughter. Her daughter, Sarah Jones, survived and married but tragically she died in a similar manner 25 years later.

- Multiple births were always dangerous for mother and children. In 1874 quads were born in the old toll house Cusop. Unfortunately only two survived.[22]

Suicide.

For those feeling under stress the River Wye sadly provided temptation. The medical officers were occasionally called to give evidence at inquests to confirm the cause of death before a verdict of death by suicide was recorded.

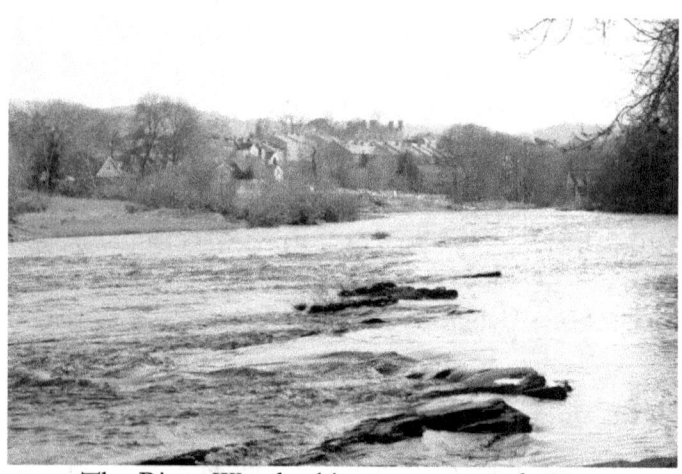

The River Wye looking west towards Hay.

Servant girl Jane Phillips was found in the river. There were no signs of a struggle, but a history of bullying by the cook at Mr Baskervilles house where Jane worked was noted.

The body of George Price a mason of Swan Bank was found floating in the river near the Warren bend after he committed suicide in June 1883.

Arthur Wobbee was the organ boy at Hay congregational church. Evidently assiduous in his duties he wore a medallion on his lapel 'Never absent, never late, Arthur Wobbee, 1908.' He worked as a gardener for Major Cockcroft at Ty-Glyn, Cusop, but following an unhappy love affair he committed suicide by drowning.

Miss Mary Powell from the Harley Almshouses went missing on the 31 December 1918. It was not until the second week in April that her body was recovered. Captain William Cornewall spotted it in the river at the corner of Old Castle Meadow Bredwardine while he was fishing. Dr Hincks testified to her identity, saying there was mental history in the family as a sister had committed suicide.[23]

Assault.

Doctors and surgeons, by the nature of their profession, were frequently called to give evidence in court cases. There are numerous reports in the papers of the Petty Sessions of the Brecon or Radnorshire Assize where they were asked to give a medical opinion on the nature of the wounds in an assault case or as to the cause of a death.

Dr Shepherd attended Albert John Wheeler when his jaw was broken by Alexander Henderson. Wheeler was working in a builder's yard when he told several children to get down from the wall of the yard for their own safety. In the process a toy train was broken. This caused Henderson to enter the yard and assault Wheeler breaking his jaw in two places. For this he was committed to the next Quarter Sessions.[24]

David James was charged with shooting and wounding John James on Llanwin Common Glasbury. The defendant admitted discharging an old pistol in the direction of the accuser because his sister objected to John James advances. He said that he had only loaded it with dust. There was no bullet. The following day John James saw Dr Bogle who said that the wounding amounted to a number of small perforations which were weeping slightly. There was no blood. After hearing evidence both parties asked to confer. They agreed no malice was intended and the doctors bill would be paid. With no evidence offered the jury returned a verdict of not guilty.[25]

Frequently courts or inquests called evidence from two doctors. It might be that a second doctor was required to confirm the diagnosis. When the patient died a second doctor would often be asked to perform the post-mortem.

A father and son named Burton were convicted of manslaughter following the violent death of William Price a respectable farmer of Clyro. The son was courting Mr Price's daughter, but her father objected. Burton, father and son, confronted the farmer and Mr Price was struck on the head and collapsed.

Mr Reece attested William Price had a weak heart and the blow was sufficient to cause the rupture discovered at the post-mortem conducted by Mr Lyde and Mr Trumper. The case was all the more poignant as Mr Reece said he had attended the Price family several times within the last few weeks due to the death of three of their children.[26]

Industrial Disease.

With a rural based economy the amount of industrial disease in Hay would have been low. There are no reports of any industrial disease concerns by the medical officers in their annual reports. Unless this caused a major outbreak it is highly unlikely that they would have reported it.

Respiratory disease is the most common. In Wales this is normally associated with coal mining but there have never been any coal mines in the Hay area. It is highly probable that there would have been Farmers Lung, a respiratory condition caused by dust in dry hay or straw.

The second most prevalent industrial disease is non-infective dermatitis, a skin disease caused by exposure to chemicals. Tanning was a major source of this. There was at least one tannery on the eastern edge of town near the Watergate, and a few cases must have occurred in the days before there was a full awareness of all the dangers of this process. The other major source of chemical use, outside a domestic setting, would be farming where other cases may have occurred.

Farming was the most important dangerous industry around Hay. It was, and still is, a continuing source of accidents but it is also responsible for a great deal of illness. Rheumatism is an occupational hazard, as is osteoarthritis due to general wear and tear from manual work.

Although farming was a major employer of manual labour most of the population would been manually employed in some capacity or another. They would all have suffered back problems from repetitive, work such as with a pick and shovel, the continual use of wheelbarrows, heavy lifting, pushing and pulling heavy boxes, field working, etc.. Women would have developed wrist or shoulder pain.

At the time rest was the only treatment available, and this was not possible in the days of 'no work no pay'.

In farming it is unlikely that brucellosis, a disease acquired from cows milk, would have been a problem to those infected. Due to its non-specific symptoms it was not widely recognised, and fatalities were rare. As late as the 1970's 30 patients a year were diagnosed with it in South-West Wales.

Inquests.

Doctors were frequently called to attend inquests to attest to the cause of death. The most common verdict for the sudden death of middle aged/elderly men in the 1860's was 'apoplexy' or '....nerves of the heart'.[27]

A typical case was the itinerant razor-grinder John Smith who died at his lodgings in Hay. Dr Bogle performed a post-mortem which confirmed death was caused by 'extravasation of blood on the brain (apoplexy)'. Current medical terminology is likely to have recorded a haemorrhagic stroke.[28]

An inquest was held on 20 March 1841 in the Vale of Glamorgan on Lewis, the eleven-year-old son of James and Mary Price, who died at the Swan Hotel in Hay. Death occurred instantaneously either by the bursting of a blood vessel or some other unexplained cause. The verdict this time was given as died by 'the visitation of god'.[29]

A particularly tragic death was recorded at the inquest of nine-year-old Alfred Thomas from Mouse Castle just outside Hay. He went out to the fields at Lower Lyde Farm to harvest vetches for Peter Burlton. When they paused for lunch Joseph Trilloe gave him two horns of cider and some bread and cheese.

Later Alfred was working with groom Henry Jenkins who acquired a jug of cider which they both drained. The boy was said not to have shown any signs of intoxication but was found later outside his house collapsed onto his face in cow muck.

Mr Lane the medical officer was called but due to a mix up was delayed in attending for which he was censured by the coroner. Alfred died from fits brought on by alcohol poisoning.[30] Given the state of the water supply it is likely that consumption of alcohol by minors was not unusual, although hopefully not in such quantities at such a tender age.

In 1925 Rosa Blanche Williams, aged 39 years, had been at Hay Market all day. Late in the afternoon she set off home to Pant Farm in the hills of Radnorshire. The weather was worsening and a snowstorm blew up as she reached Painscastle. The landlord of the Maesllwch Inn, William Morgan, beseeched her to stay the night till the storm had passed.

Rosa said she was anxious to get home to her six children, one of whom she was nursing. She set off up the hill behind the inn but sadly the storm proved too fierce and she died within a few hundred yards on Rhulen Hill. Her pony had thrown her in the raging blizzard. At the inquest Dr Hincks said her ankle was swollen but not broken and the verdict was she died 'due to syncope following exposure'.

It is possible Rosa had broken her midfoot, an injury difficult to diagnose without the benefit of an X-ray. (For fuller details of this incident see Appendix 1 page 201).

Another potential peril.

An unusual incident was recorded by Bramwell Bradley, an orphan who came to Hay to live with his grandparents in Bear Street. Bramwell was first employed as kitchen boy at Hay Castle in 1925 before going on to be the hall porter. The etiquette of the time was that he could not be called a butler, although that was his role, because the castle had no footmen.

Bramwell's mother Maud had married Harold Bradley in 1912. Unfortunately Harold died in 1918 after being hit by a train while walking home with a sack on his back.

Bramwell recalled how his grandmother Emma remembered Harold in his coffin. He felt warm to the touch and his flesh bounced back. This was so unlike other family members Emma visited in later life when she went to pay her respects.

As she got older Emma feared that Harold may have been in a deep coma, not dead, and was buried alive. She though that in the early 19th century the doctors may not have detected a faint heartbeat. She always had her children and grandchildren promise to put a mirror under her nose to make sure she was dead before she was buried.[31]

Notes.
[1] Anonymous, Medical Practice in Radnorshire, *Transactions of the Radnorshire Society* (1933) 27–35.
[2] *Hereford Times* (11 September 1858).
[3] *Hereford Times* (2 November 1850).
[4] *Hereford Journal* (13 October 1852).
[5] *Brecon County Times* (27 November 1913).
[6] *Brecon County Times* (19 December 1868).
[7] *Hereford Times* (20 March 1852).
[8] *Brecon County Times* (22 August 1868).
[9] *Cardiff Times* (July 1884).
[10] *Cardiff Times* (Oct 1876).
[11] *Brecon County Times* (11 Augustn1866).
[12] *Brecon County Times* (7 August 1869).
[13] *Hereford Journal* (2 November 1859).
[14] *Hereford Times* (9 April 1853).
[15] *Brecon County Times* (23 April 1909).
[16] *Hereford Journal* (14 December 1853).
[17] *Kington Times* (15 December 1928).
[18] *Hereford Times* (10 August 1850).
[19] *Hereford Journal* (25 July and 1 August 1863).
[20] *Brecon County Times* (March 1916).
[21] Hore-Ruthven, Elyned, A Victorian Childhood, in Lewis, Colin, *Under the Black Mountains: The History of Gwernyfed since 1600*, Logaston Press (2017) 60.
[22] *Monmouthshire Merlin* (16 October 1874).
[23] *Brecon County Times* (17 April 1919).
[24] *Brecon County Times* (7 October 1915).
[25] *Hereford Journal* (9 August 1862).
[26] *Hereford Journal* (12 May 1858.)
[27] *Brecon County Times* (15 June 1867).
[28] *Brecon County Times* (20 October 1866).
[29] *Cardiff and Merthyr Guardian, Glamorgan, Monmouth, and Brecon Gazette* (20 March 1841).
[30] *Hereford Times* (2 July 1859).
[31] Mrs Ann Hitchcox family tradition.

Chapter 4 – Public Health

According to Gerald of Wales,[1] the 13th century chronicler who lived near Brecon, the area around Hay was bountiful. It produced a great deal of corn, the pastures were full of cattle, and woodland full of wildlife. The Rivers Usk and Wye were teeming with freshwater fish, trout and salmon, and the Wye particularly bountiful with grayling. Brecknock Mere, also known as Clamosus but now as Llangorse Lake, had pike, perch, trout, tench and eels.

With this abundance of natural resources it could be expected that the inhabitants of Hay would have been healthier than those in crowded urban areas. Unfortunately this was not necessarily so. There were a multitude of other factors influencing public health. In past times life was precarious and people often died very young.

Sanitation was poor, water often polluted, food hygiene non-existent, and storage systems for food during the winter months led to gastrointestinal problems. It is attention to these matters, rather than medical advances, that have led to the greatest improvements in the general health of the population. This applied in Hay as much as it did elsewhere.

Population of Hay.

Assessing population numbers in medieval times is largely educated guess work. One measure is based on the number of burgage plots. These were the long narrow gardens or parcels of land stretching out behind the houses and shops of high streets in medieval towns. Over centuries they have often remained relatively unchanged and have been used to estimate population numbers fairly accurately.

In Hay it has been estimated that, based on these plots, there were approximately 400 inhabitants in 1340 before the Black Death.

Subsequent populations can be estimated from a formula based on birth rates, and again these have proved to be generally accurate.

Figures are far more accurate since the introduction of the national census.

Year	Population
1340	400
1690	455
1715	444
1725	771
1760	750
1780	838
1800	873
1810	1210
1820	1050
1840	1410

Census Year	Population
1801	822
1830	1455
1851	1952
1861	1997
1911	1603
1921	1533
1991	1407

Child mortality rates in Victorian times for those under 5 years of age do not make pleasant reading. The rates in Hay were no different to other areas.

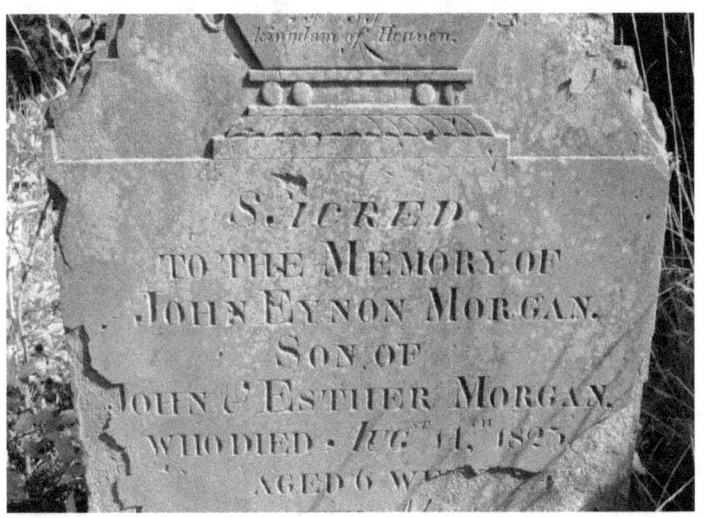

A grave marker for a child only 6 weeks old in St Marys churchyard.

Without the benefit of modern medicine childhood ailments such as measles, whooping cough, poliomyelitis, diphtheria and scarlet fever were often fatal. If you survived to five years of age you had a good chance that you would make adulthood.

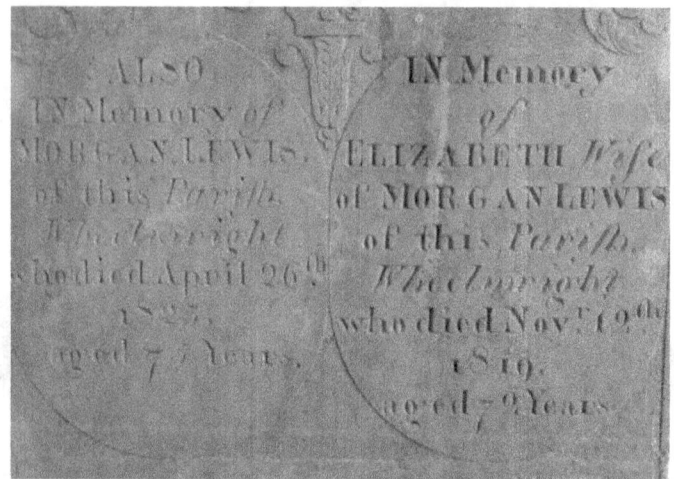

Two parishioners in St Mary's churchyard who lived to a ripe old age.

The parish registers show mortality figures for children of between 26.5% and 38.5% between 1801 and 1840. These were down from 50-60% in the 1750's, caused by a combination of the insanitary conditions and disease.

The Medical Officer (M.O.) of Health's Annual Report for 1856 reported there were 47 deaths, with 12 under 1yr and 14 over 60yrs, and 73 births with 42 female and 31 male. There were several epidemics of measles (which was fairly normal) but no other infectious diseases. The sanitary conditions of the town were 'much as usual'.

In 1859 there were 34 births and 30 deaths, [2] and the report for 1885 identified 51 deaths, only 1 from typhoid fever, and 79 births.

Although life spans could be short they were not for everyone and many people lived full lifespans of three score years and ten.

Vestry Committees.

From medieval times every parish had a Vestry Committee. Their role evolved and developed from the feudal system. Initially they only administered the running of the church and appointment of its officers. Gradually they also took on the supervision of civic affairs. This included law enforcement, support for the poor, suppression of vagrancy, maintenance of roads and control of vermin, etc..

Their multitude of roles, and the increasing movement of persons as a result of industrialisation, led to committees becoming overwhelmed. In particular supervision and support for the poor was neglected.

As time went on sub committees called Select Vestries developed to undertake aspects of civic affairs.

Board of Guardians Hay Union.

The Select Committees became more and more corrupt and as a result the 1834 Poor Law Amendment Act was brought in. This allowed the setting up of Boards of Guardians from 1836 to supervise civic affairs and the care of the poor. Crucially they were responsible for the building and running of Workhouses.

Boards were composed of members who represented each of the parishes of the Workhouse Unions. In the case of Hay Union there was one from each parish, with two from the largest centres of population, at Hay and Pwll-y-wrach. Boards also appointed a supernumerary vicar and medical officer.

Mr Caple was the first medical appointee, but he must have resigned almost before he took up his post as an advertisement for his replacement was dated 1838.[3] This was just two years after the board was set up, and only one year after the tenders for building and fitting out of the workhouse were placed.

An advertisement in 1842 shows the area the M.O. covered - Hay, Llanigon, Bredwardine, Clifford, Cusop, Dorstone, Whitney, Bryngwyn, Clyro, Llanbedr Painscastle, Llandenyfach and Llowes. In addition he was also responsible for the Workhouse. The post offered a salary of £85 to include all medicines.[4]

The Local Government Board.

Although for centuries people thought that contagious diseases were caught from bad smells or 'miasmas' as they were known no one thought to try and eradicate the causes of them. In many cases they were made worse by such acts as emptying 'night soil' from chamber pots directly into the street.

As we have seen there was no clear understanding of the role of good sanitation in preventing the major cholera epidemics in the early 1800's. Nevertheless due to this Local Boards were set up nationally in 1848 with specific responsible for sanitation and public health. Their remit included water supplies, drainage, cleaning, abattoirs, and burial grounds.

Boards comprised nine members elected by the male householders of the town, again with a supernumerary doctor and vicar. Salaried officers were appointed to support them.

In Hay the Board was concerned about the grossly insanitary state of much of the housing, although in all probability this was no worse than elsewhere. That there was ongoing concern is indicated by the letter to the Hereford Times in 1853 complaining about the filthy state of the town.[5]

The Board took its duties seriously even to the extent of taking three residents to court because they had not complied with an order to provide sufficient 'troughing to their houses to prevent rainwater falling on the pavement' i.e., guttering.[6]

In 1840 there were only 305 houses in the town. By 1863 the population had increased by about a third, but there was no corresponding increase in housing. The new waterworks had opened but it was reported that 104 houses still had an inadequate water supply. Drainage also appears to have been a recurrent issue as the 1856 Medical Officer of Health's Annual Report stated drainage was 'as usual'.

Typical of the concerns they addressed was the summonsing of George Wood, a shoemaker. He kept pigs in his house, and as a result they thought it 'not being in a wholesome and cleanly state'.

In 1878 proceedings were taken against William Arter of High Town. He was a Marine Storekeeper i.e. dealer in rags, bones, rabbit skins, and possibly a fishmonger. He was prohibited from using his house for habitation.

The streets were also a concern. Every week a pig market was held around the Police Station (the present St Johns Chapel and restaurant). In 1873 Sir Joseph E. Bailey, the Lord of the Manor, was requested to flag or pave this area to enable it to be kept clean.

The importance of good sanitation began to be recognised, if not understood. The severe outbreak of scarlet fever that occurred in 1880 was attributed to the insanitary conditions in the town.

Medical Officers.

Despite recognition of the need for improvements support for the meetings of the Board was poor, with an average attendance of only 50%.

The Board was supposed to have a Medical Officer of Health but there was a delay. The first appointment was not until 1868. This was a joint appointment covering Hay and parts of Radnorshire. A separate officer was appointed to cover Radnorshire from 1912.[7]

How seriously the medical officers took their duties is difficult to say. Dr Shepherd never attended a meeting of the Board and few stayed in post for long, possibly because the remuneration was poor.

The appointed medical officers were:

1868 Dr Henry Proctor. No salary.
1872 Surgeon Mr E. Smith.
1876 Dr Giles at £1. 1s. 0d. per day.
1878 Dr Clouston at £5pa.
1880 Dr Appleby.
1886 Dr Shepherd.
1897 Dr T.G. Dickson.
1899 Dr G.W.B. Featherstone.

There was a distinct change in 1901 with the appointment of Dr Tom Hincks. He was paid £20pa and initially stayed in post until 1910. On the 7 August that year the Urban District Council confirmed his reappointed but with a stipend of only £5 per annum. However in addition he was allowed a fee of £1.17s.6d for each patient.[8]

Urban District Councils.

The Local Boards were superseded by Urban District Councils in 1894, again with nine representatives and similar responsibilities.

The Boards and later the Councils were required to supervise lodging houses to ensure there was no overcrowding.

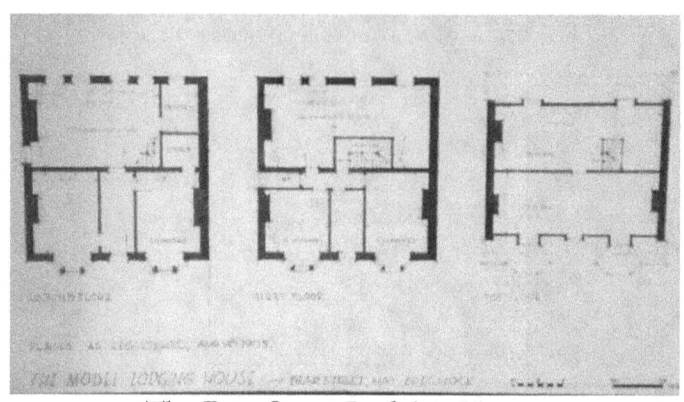
The Bear Street Lodging House.

The Council approved an application by Mr John Greenway for 39 lodgers in a purpose-built house at the top of Bear Street. This had 5 bedrooms - 2 with 9 male lodgers each, 1 with 5 lodgers and another with 4 lodgers. A large room held space for 12 lodgers who were married couples. It was noted that there was 'provision of partitions between beds occupied by married couples'. Licenses were also issued to two houses in Chancery Lane, for 8 and 10 lodgers, and two in Heol y Dwr, for 22 and 21 lodgers.

Many of the Council's main concerns continued year on year and were highlighted in the medical officers annual report. In April 1913 Dr Tom Hincks reported he had examined two cases of tuberculosis in the district. He also confirmed that Dr Bridge the County Medical Officer had checked the water supply following a visit to the waterworks and was very dissatisfied with the standard of the water as he had found manure close to the stream.

On the standard of housing Dr Bridge was also unhappy, reporting that at least one of the houses he had seen was not fit for human habitation. A councillor Mr Sidney Williams added that it was not the only one as many others were just as bad.

Water Supply.

For centuries the people of Hay collected water from the seven public well-springs.

- Town Well at the bottom of Ship Pitch is near the steps by the path leading south along the old town walls. It is now dry and currently marked by a square stone in the wall. This was the site of the medieval gateway through the town walls known as the Watergate.
- Black Lion Well on Black Lion Green is the trickle of water in the angle of the Dulas Brook below the houses on the left. Legend has it that whichever of a newly married couple drinks first from the well will wear the trousers in the marriage. A traditional tale has a groom hurrying off to the well straight after the wedding ceremony. As he did so his bride opened her purse and produced a bottle of spring water that she had collected the previous day.
- St Johns Well, also called Castle Well, was in Oxford Road, set in the wall surrounding the castle lawns. Charles Portman[9] described it as opposite the path from Caemar but the exact site was lost when the collapsed garden wall was rebuilt.

- Swan Well is the gem of the well-springs in Hay.

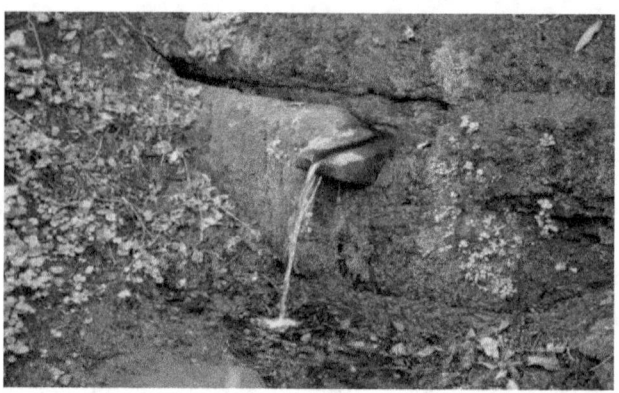

The well is clearly visible as a pretty stream of water flowing from a channel on the west side of the path along the Login Brook behind the Harley Almshouses. The stream has never been known to stop running either in the driest of summers or in the severest of winters.

During the hot summer of 1976 farmers would fill containers of water for their animals. To this day it is often possible to see vehicles stop in the road by the gate opposite the church and go down to collect a supply of this crystal clear nectar for their own consumption.

- St Marys Well is in the garden of Sackville Cottage.

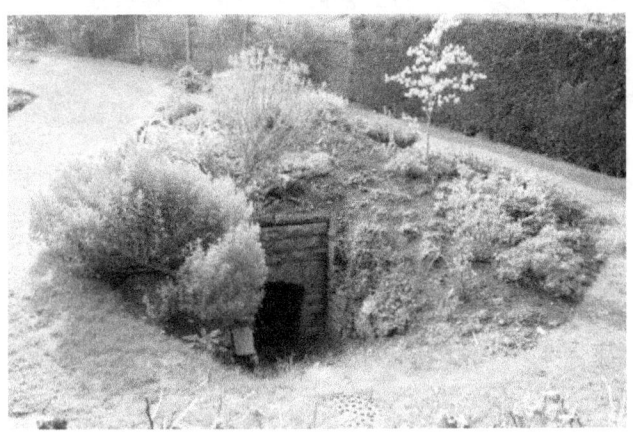

Behind the tower in St Mary's churchyard an arched opening is visible in the facing garden. Now dry, reputedly a spout of water from it dowsed a fire in the tower during its rebuild in 1834.
- Eye Well is on the riverbank below the path leading to the Warren. Small with a poor flow but reputedly with medicinal properties for treating eye ailments. Whether incantations are necessary as the water is collected, as required at the spring in Rock Gardens Llandrindod Wells, is not known.[10]
- Walk Well lies below Eye Well at the river's edge. A trickle of water seeps from the riverbank through a tangle of moss into a stone trough on the historic stone quay. This is reputed to have been built for the barges from Hereford bringing stone to build the church. It was more likely to have been one side

of a ferry crossing, the quay on the other side of the River Wye having now washed away.

The 1890 Guide to Hay has a section about the river walk. It says that near the church:

'an inclined path leads down to the Walk Well, a perennial fountain of purest spring water flowing from a lichen clothed rock upon the river bank; a source from whence many of the inhabitants are provided with water for the table; and to the left of the path above referred to, now almost hidden by the bramble and rough herbage covering the slope, is a tiny spring called the Eye Well which in olden times was famed for its virtues in curing diseases of the eye.'[1]

In addition to the well-springs there are a number of private wells in the town, including one in the grounds of a cafe, one in the yard of no. 2 Castle Street, and another in the grounds of the old workhouse. Rock House, the old gas board showroom, has one in its cellar.

By Victorian times the wells were becoming polluted by the local cesspits and night soil buckets. Eventually in 1863, due to the lobbying of Henry Allen of Oakfield, reservoirs were built on Hay Common and piped into town. On 30 October of that year it was reported in the Hereford Journal that there was a dispute by Mr Bayliss, the contractor, over monies owed. The directors of the Waterworks Company paid him after he reduced the amount of his claim.

An extra strain on supplies occurred with the opening of the Brecon to Hereford Railway. This opened in stages from 1863 but it was not until the

Midland Railway took it over in 1874 that it came into its heyday. As the line became busier the importance of a pure supply of water assumed greater prominence. The quality of the water from the Black Hills meant engines routinely stopped at Hay to top up their tanks.

Increasing demand led to the reservoirs being enlarged in 1867, and additional water was piped into them from the Dulas Brook high in the dingle above Cusop. The following year was very dry and the supply failed. As a result inhabitants had to resort to their wells or the water carriers who brought water up from the river.[12]

Keen to preserve supplies and prevent waste the reservoir company policed the responsible use of its supply. In July 1868 the company took Andrew Bridges, a marine store dealer i.e. a dealer in rabbit fur, rags and bones, to court. He had allowed the tap in his premises to be turned on for a considerable length of time and so wasted water. He was fined 6 shillings.[13]

The flow of water from these reservoirs was said to be good in 1877 but by 1885 there was an insufficient supply during the summer months. Encouragingly when samples were submitted to Professor Wanklyn of London in 1886 he stated that they showed the water was 'Organically pure and free from sewerage matter'.

Over time the pipes corroded further reducing the supply. To alleviate this an additional supply was provided in 1887 by piping a spring into a reservoir at Llangwathen, the ancient farmhouse beside the Dulas Brook in Cusop.

Despite this it was only a few years later in the 1890s that the supply once again became erratic. In 1895 the town was without water for a period of 8 weeks, with little attempt to repair the pipes. The following year the Urban District Council bought the water company for a sum of £3,330.

Despite the councils oversight an irregular water supply was a continuing problem. As late as 1903 the Rev. de Winton recorded that he put cattle on the glebe land near Hay church to provide milk for his family as he was unsure of the safety of the local water supply.[14]

In 1912 the supply failed due to an airlock necessitating the installation of air valves to prevent recurrence before the key summer months.

Dr Tom Hincks questioned the quality of the water supply in his 1913 Medical Officer of Health's Annual Report. As a result later that year the Board resolved to clean out the filter beds in the reservoirs on the common. To do so meant a break in the supply to the town for two weeks. Again they resolved to secure an additional supply into the reservoir at Llangwathen to cover the break.[15]

An indication of the water consumption can be gained from the report of the quantity used during the first half of 1908 - 3,345,000 gallons out of the company's yearly limit of 6,000,000.[16]

The problem was so acute that at one stage a Council Chairman Alderman Like made a proposal that the old castle mott be used as a reserve supply.

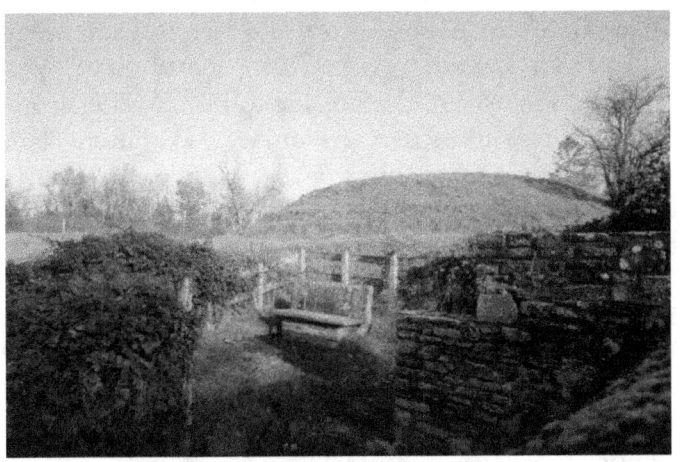

The Tump near St Mary's Church.

He suggested that the inside of the Tump, as it is known locally, be scooped out, brick lined and filled with water as a reserve supply. This would save the legs of the Town Crier 'Bumper' Howells who had to declare any cut in supply.

In the 1930's the supply was so bad that the town surveyor Billy Morgans investigated and found more water ran to waste than was consumed. The sound of water running underground could be heard in High Town, reputedly coming from the pipes created from tree trunks. Despite this, predictably, Councillor Like's proposal came to nothing.[17]

The water supplies continued to be erratic. The town was subject to water shortages in the summer of 1953 when the water would be cut off twice a day to allow supplies to replenish. Approaches were made to Major Booth of Cusop who had a plentiful source of water from a spring on his land. Unfortunately he refused to allow the fire brigade to pump water from his source to the reservoirs on Hay Common. The solution was for the fire brigade to make night-time clandestine visits to Cusop Dingle and pump water all the way from the Dulas Brook to the common.

Lord Glanusk as Lord of the Manor of Hay had rights over the common where the reservoirs had been constructed. On his death in 1950 his executors relinquished all rights to the common, and the reservoirs and waterworks on it, to the Urban District Council.[18]

Public Houses.

A common misconception is that polluted water supplies meant that until relatively recent times it was safer to drink alcoholic beverages than to drink water. This was not necessarily so.

Medieval settlements grew up around fresh running water, a spring or a well. This may be refreshing but in the absence of tea or coffee the population looked for an alternative flavoured drink.

Small beer was popular with both adults and children This was a low-calorie low alcohol ale made by fermenting barley rather than hops with yeast. It was viewed to be more beneficial than ordinary beer to workers and farmers in need of energy.

As a result there were numerous licensed premises, and Slaters Directory of 1864 listed 32 in Hay. The town was renowned for the number it had.

Name.	Owner.	Location
Traveller's Trap .	Gwynne.	Lion Street.
The Sun.	Gorst.	4 Brecon Rd.
The Old Oak.	Crompton.	Royal Oak?
(possibly Golden Oak House, Brecon Road)		
The Swan.	Unknown.	11 Church St.
Royal George.	Unknown.	15? Castle St.
Blue Boar.	Unknown.	16 Castle St.
The White Cock	Edwards.	12 Castle St?
Grapes.	Gittens.	
Golden Lion.	Unknown.	21 Castle St.
(Madigan's original cycle shop).		
The Dog, then Talbot.	E.M. Lloyd.	5 Castle St.

Name	Proprietor	Address
Mason's Arms. (now the Spar Supermarket).	Unknown.	26 Castle St.
The Fountain.	A.S. Williams.	
Market Tavern.	A. Williams.	Castle Square.
The Bell.	T. Pugh.	Bell Bank.
The Bear.	T. Price.	1 Bear St.
New Inn.	A. Powell.	Bear St.
Black Lion.	Unknown.	26 Lion St.
Drovers Arms.	Mrs W. Turner.	
Half Moon.	Unknown.	37 Lion St.
Castle Inn.	H. Batts.	
Wheat Sheaf.	Unknown.	38 Lion St.
Red Lion.	Tom Pugh.	41 Lion St.
Old Mitre.	Robert Williams.	
Kings Head.	T. Wright.	
The Rose and Crown.	Unknown.	10 Broad St.
Three Tuns.	Unknown.	4 Broad St.
Black Swan.	George Price.	5 Broad St.
The Seven Stars	Unknown.	11 Broad St.
Tanners Arms.	M. Jones.	31 Broad St.
Ship.	J. Smith.	Newport St.
The Lamb.	Unknown.	Wyeford Rd.
Bridge-End.	G.A. Lage.	41 Newport St.

In addition, there were another dozen or so in the town at some stage e.g. Old White Lion Broad Street, Three Horse Shoes 7 High Town, Wine Vaults 12 Castle Street, Cock Inn 12 Castle Street, New Sun 3 Brecon Road. The King's Arms may have been another name for the Rose and Crown. Often these were little more than tap rooms in the front parlour of houses.

There is no record that there was a particular problem with alcohol abuse in Hay. Nevertheless the various friendly societies, with the Salvation Army and the vicar of Hay the Rev. William Latham Bevan, worked hard to reduce alcohol consumption.

This work continued after the Rev. Bevans death. Ironically a temperance group met in the upper rooms of the Wheatsheaf Inn, Lion Street, into the 1920's. There was also a Temperance Hotel at the top of Castle Street, and this continued into the 1970's.

This relatively high number of licensed premises continued into the 20th century. The police licencing authorities objected to a licence renewal in 1934 because there were already 19 pubs in town. This was one public house per 126 head of population compared to one per 526 generally in Wales.

The true extent of drunkenness or illness due to drink is unknown. It is possible that not being able to open on a Sunday due to the Sunday Closing Act between 1881 and the acts repeal in 1969 helped keep it under control.

At one time there was another licenced premise. The Nelson (now Kingfisher House) was just over the English border in Cusop near Hay railway station. As it was not in Wales it was not subject to Sunday closing but voluntarily followed the Welsh legislation to prevent local ill feeling.

Lt Col. Harry Llewellyn of Foxhunter fame, and the chairman of Badgers Brewery, drew the first pint on its first Sunday opening in 1969.

Drainage.

In addition to the problems with the intermittent water supply there was no proper sewage or refuse disposal system in the town for a long time. Even disposal of the dead was largely unrecorded.

For many years one of the main town sewers discharged into the Login Brook. This was an open water leat at the bottom of the hill where Church Street meets Brecon Road. Indeed the name Login means dirty water, possibly shortened from Halogyn meaning the polluted one.[19]

The Urban District Council minutes of 6 January 1896 noted a letter from Hereford Town Council alleging pollution of the River Wye by sewage from Hay. Eventually in February 1898 a town committee replied and provided reasons to continue the existing sewerage arrangements.

- Matters have been so from 'time immemorial' and no epidemic has been traced to it.
- There is 30 miles of fast flowing gravely river between Hay and Hereford.
- Villages in between Hay and Hereford also discharge into the river.
- The committee also noted that Hereford itself discharged sewerage into the river above the city.

It was only a few years later in 1904 that Lord Tredegar complained about the state of the Login Brook. He paid for the ugly sewer pipe still to be seen to be laid in the bed of the brook. It discharged directly into the Wye. This was an improvement but was not thought to be entirely satisfactory. A committee was formed in 1905 to enquire into arrangements in other towns.

Inevitably things moved slowly as considerable finance was potentially involved. Eventually in February 1914 a site was leased from Henry Sheen for a sewerage scheme. The council held the project over, and in April 1916 costs of £125.15s.7d. were settled with no other action.[20] A proper foul water treatment plant was not installed until 1969 at the other end of town at the Gliss.

Also at the other end of town were the mills and forges of the industrial complex at Ship Pitch. Here they were separately served by the open water leat which ran along Heol y Dwr. This had a long history. It ran from the upper reaches of the Dulas Brook across the fields and through Hay before draining into the River Wye. At one stage it supplied a leather-bottle factory in Heol y Dwr.

There must have been recurrent issues with this supply or drainage.In his 1886 Annual Medical Report Dr Hincks stated that the drainage in Heol y Dwr was improved.

Refuse disposal in the town was formalised in 1895. A contract for five shillings a week was given to William Lilwall, a.k.a. the Scavenger, to collect dust and sweepings from the streets, along with household ashes. These were all dumped in the Wye together with household refuse. This led to further complaints from residents in Hereford, who received the refuse in due course.

The refuse was collected by horse and cart and in the 1890's the horse was called Mazeppa. Apparently, it had a ferocious appetite for oats and was costing the ratepayers a fortune. A two-man sub-committee was formed to investigate. It found that the unfortunate animal was kept indoors summer and winter instead of being turned out to pasture. There is no official record that this situation was remedied, or the fate of the unusually named Mazeppa.

The duties of Mazeppa and the Scavenger included taking the council water cart around the streets at times of water shortages. The role of Scavenger also involved turning the valves of the reservoirs on and off as necessary.

Leisure Amenities.

As living conditions improved at the end of the Victorian era people began to have the time and money to participate in increased leisure activities. The value of open air and exercise was increasingly recognised.

The Warren field, in the crook of the River Wye on the western edge of town, was a free amenity enjoyed by the general population for generations.

This was the site of the Hay Golf Club when a 9-hole course was opened in 1903. Mr F.A. Goss a professional from Hereford laid it out although it was slightly short at 1,865 yards. The president Hon. H.C. Devereux reported in 1921 that it had been extended to a full 9 holes. It seems that the short holes were extended so that the course became full length.

The beautiful location enhanced it as a popular pastime, particularly as from its inception the club admitted ladies and junior members. Many of its members were the most prominent citizens of the town.[21]

The club largely owed its existence to C.E. Tunnard-Moore of Cusop, the Vicar of Hay Rev. J.J. de Winton and Arthur Chapman.

In 1910 the luminaries were the Hon R.C. Devereaux as president, with Maj. W.H. Booth D.S.O., Capt. W. de Winton, Capt. Glen Kidston, Col. R.D. Garnons-Williams, Revs. G. Leigh Spencer and H. W. Trumper, and Messrs W.F. Burton, E.H. Cheese, E.F. Cockcroft, H. Graystone, S. Mavrojani and H.B.C. Whitehouse as vice-presidents. Membership cost 12s6d with family tickets £1.5s.

The club played for the Savigear Cup each year until 1910. This was replaced by the Greystone Cup in 1913. Photographer and stationer H.R. Grant was a very enthusiastic member, and won the cup in 1913, 1917 and again in 1930. He won the Blackstad cup outright in 1925, one of a number of cups and bowls members played for. Others were the Presidents Cup, the Littley Cup for ladies, and the Hay Golf Club bowl. The club moved to Hay Common in 1930.

The Warren came under threat during the 1970's when there was the possibility of a caravan park being sited there. The town responded by 200 concerned citizens forming the Warren Club. This raised enough money to purchase the field and preserve it as an open space for the enjoyment of everyone. The club is still in existence, now with 300 members, who subscribe annually to maintain the Warren for general enjoyment.

A series of sporting clubs were formed in addition to the golf club.

The Hay Gymnasium was founded in 1890 with the aim to 'exercise the youth of the town in their muscles as well as their brains'. It is not known where it normally met but the third annual display and assault-at-arms was held in the Drill Hall. It had a varied programme which included Swedish Drill, rings, parallel and horizontal bars, and the vaulting horse.[22] Their annual general meetings were held in the Crown Hotel[23] as were many others such as the golf club.

It is not known when the St Mary's Football Club was formed but it played for the Club Hay Challenge Cup in the 1920's and is still in existence. By 1895 cricket and tennis clubs had also been formed.

For those with a more musical interest the town had an orchestral band in 1893, in addition to the various bands of the friendly societies.

Hay was always the recruiting ground for the men of 'D' company Brecknock Volunteer Battalion South Wales Borderers. A full company of 117 men was difficult to find following the army reorganisation in 1908 but a troop of 80 to 90 men was accepted as sufficient to maintain 'D' company in the town.

Captain Cheese, the local solicitor, was in charge in 1895, succeeded by Dr T. Hincks.

A miniature rifle range was built to support their drills, and the annual training camps. It was behind the Drovers Arms near the Drill Hall and opened by the Hon. Mrs R.C. Devereux on 9 November 1906.

Notes.
[1] Gerald of Wales, *The Journey through Wales* and *The Description of Wales*, trans by Lewis Thorpe, Penguin (1978).
[2] *The Welshman* (1 December 1859).
[3] *Hereford Journal* (14 February 1838).
[4] [4] *Silurian, Cardiff, Merthyr, and Brecon Mercury* (29 January 1842).
[5] *Hereford Times* (15 October 1853).
[6] *Brecon County Times* (19 December 1868).
[7] *Brecon County Times* (11 April 1912).
[8] Fairs, Geoffrey, *The History of Hay*, Phillimore (Chichester, 1972).
[9] Portman, Charles G.,*The Sacred Stones, Sacred Trees and Holy Wells of Hay, and the Neighbourhood*, Grant (Hay, 1907).
[10] Palmer, Roy, *Folklore of Radnorshire*, Logaston Press (2001).
[11] Grant, H.R., *Guide to Hay,* Grant Publishing (1890).
[12] *Brecon County Times* (15 August 1868).
[13] *Brecon County Times* (22 August 1868).
[14] Fairs, Geoffrey, *The History of Hay,* Phillimore (Chichester, 1972).
[15] *Brecon County Times* (6 November 1913)
[16] *Radnor Express* (16 July 1908).
[17] Marwood, Cyril, Wisps of Hay with other chaff, Arthur Stockwell (no date).
[18] Nicholls, Alan J., *Historical Directory of Hay on Wye. Rural Parish* (Lulu, 2016).
[19] Davies, John, *A History of Wales*, Penguin (1990).
[20] Fairs, Geoffrey, *The History of Hay*, Phillimore (1972)
[21] *Brecon County Times* (8 April 1910).
[22] *Brecon County Times* (31 March 1893).
[23] *Brecon County Times* (6 October 1893).

Chapter 5 – Clinical Services

To support the work of the doctors a range of other services gradually developed to serve the health needs of the inhabitants of Hay.

Dentistry.

During the Middle Ages dentistry was in the hands of the barber surgeons. There was even a dental textbook, admittedly in German, published in 1530 by Artzney Buchlein.

Gradually professional dentistry began to develop in the 18th and 19th centuries, with the first dental school opening in America in 1840. The first British dental school, the Royal Dental Hospital of London, opened in 1858.

Little is known about early dentistry in Hay but examples from around the area give an indication of the service patients could expect.

In 1838 a dental surgeon, A. Byes from Hereford, advertised the virtues of his Anodyne Cement for restoring 'Decayed Teeth' without pain, heat or pressure. He was also able to affix artificial teeth without removing the stumps of old teeth – a single tooth 10s. and a complete set on an 18-carat gold plate for £20.[1]

In those early days dentists often travelled to neighbouring towns to provide a clinic. From one we can get a good indication of the costs. Mr J.J. Sylvester, Surgeon Dentist from Worcester, regularly visited Kington in 1848. His advertised charges were:

Stopping teeth: each tooth 5s to 10s.
Filling teeth: each tooth 2s 6d to 5s.
Sealing the teeth: each tooth 5s to 10s.
Extraction of permanent teeth each tooth 5s.
Extraction of primary teeth: each tooth 2s 6d.
Insertion of teeth, on gold plate: from £1 to £1 10s.[2]

The good Mr Sylvester also warned about using camphor compound as a dentifrice (toothpaste). In a letter to the Hereford Journal he warned that it had the unfortunate effect of 'causing the enamel to become friable, rendering decay at the neck of the teeth, but also effecting a recession of the gums'.[3]

From about 1860 Messrs Levason and Robertson surgeon dentists of Bridge Street, Hereford began advertising a clinic on alternate Fridays in the Swan Hotel in Hay. This may also have been where Rev. Francis Kilvert saw the 'new anaesthetic' laughing gas on St Swithin's day 1871.

With no resident dentist in the town, emergency dental work was done by the local doctors. In 1872 the Rev. Francis Kilvert mentions calling Dr Coulson to treat an infected tooth.

It was not until 1919 after the First World War that Henderson's Dental Surgery opened in Brooke House, Hay. It advertised every branch of dentistry, all hours daily.[4]

After the Second World War James M. Brookes set up a dental practice at Wye View 25/26 Broad Street on Thursdays 9-4. This was taken over and became Wilsons the dentist.

Mr Wilson's wife did not trust her husband's driving so always hired a car to take her to Hereford. Mr Wilson drove a small car, a Standard 8 or 10, with a sunshine roof. Being quite tall he would often drive along the Hardwick Road into Hay with his head sticking out of the top of the car.[5]

Siege of Lion Street.

Dentistry provided a memorable incident in more recent times. What became known as the Siege of Lion Street occurred in the first-floor dental surgery at 43 Lion Street on 10 December 1994.

Edward Mark Williams held ten patients and staff hostage for fifteen hours armed with what turned out to be an imitation firearm. The police and S.A.S. soldiers from Hereford besieged the building overnight, but in the event Williams was overpowered peaceably by the hostages. They talked and talked until the gunman fell asleep. The local vet, Ros Coles, then walked over and relieved him of his gun, whereupon four others grabbed him.[6]

A Tragic case of Toothache.

The 'cure all' ingredient arsenic was also used in dentistry. Mixed with creosote and morphine it was used to treat toothache.

This combination may have been known to Emma Bevan, an 18-year-old servant at the Bear Inn in Bear Street. When she developed a tooth infection she retired to bed after taking Spirit of Oil, now known as creosote. The following morning she was discovered dead. On her bedside table was an empty bottle of Spirits of Salt, also called Muriatic acid but now known as hydrochloric acid.

The inquest made no mention of arsenic. Emma may not have had time to purchase any, or no one thought to enquire if she had. The coroner recorded a verdict of accidental death due to the effects of the two substances.[7]

Nursing Services.

The derivation of the word nurse in Latin means 'I nourish' and from the earliest times men and women in religious orders attended to the sick. With the demise of the religious houses from the 16th century a relative or neighbour might care for the infirm.

Formal nursing training started in 1860 in London, but it was not until 1919 that nursing registration was established. Before then nurse was the generic term for anyone employed to look after babies and infants, ill adults or the elderly sick.

Any training necessary would have occurred 'on the job' by assisting someone more experienced.

The census returns from 1851 to 1901 give an indication of the large number of persons calling themselves nurses employed in Hay.

- Catherine Herbert (aged 66 in 1851) – nurse living at 5 Gravel Lane. In 1861 and 1871 she was living at Bell Bank.
- Catherine Herbert (aged 24 in 1851) (daughter of the above?) – nurse employed at 6 Horse Fair (Hay Castle!) to look after Mary E. the four-month-old daughter of Rev. William L. Bevan.
- Ruth Williams (aged 53 in 1851) – nurse lived at Royal Oak Row. By 1871 she had retired and was living at 17 Brecon Road (possibly the same house).

- Ann Thomas (aged 10 in 1861) – nurse at 2 Wernllwyn to one year old William and a four-hour old infant daughter, the children of William Davies, shepherd.
- Ann Warton (aged 13 in 1861) – nurse at the Black Lion Inn to look after Steven the nine-month-old son of the innkeeper John Allen.
- Hannah Williams (aged 51 in 1861) – widowed nurse living at Cwmdwydwr, Cusop.
- Elizabeth Smith (aged 51 in 1861) – employed as hospital nurse at the Workhouse.
- Jane Jones (aged 17 in 1861) – nurse at 49 Broad Street caring for eleven-month-old Clara daughter of William Webb the miller.

- Sylva Lewis (aged 57 in 1871) – widowed retired nurse lodging at 42 Lion Street. In 1861 she had been living in the Gwynne Almshouse at 2 Chain Alley with her husband John.
- Emily Smith (aged 25 in 1871) – nursemaid at 11 Oxford Road to Mary the eight-month-old daughter of surgeon Dr Joseph Smith.
- Anne Meredith (aged 24 in 1871) – employed as a nurse at 5 Church Street by bank accountant James Griffiths to look after his one-year-old daughter Fortune.
- Maria Parnell (aged 17 in 1871) – nurse at 9 Church Street to the young family of George Page solicitor.
- Georgina Portman (aged 64 in 1871) – nurse and head of her household at 14 Brecon Rd.
- Elizabeth Williams (aged 62 in 1871) – nurse to residents in Harleys Almshouses in Brecon Road.

- Hannah Evans (aged 16 in 1881) – nurse at Compton House 1 High Town to one year old Ellen daughter of Henry Stephens, draper.

- Annie M. Newman (aged 14 in 1891) – nurse at 5 Oxford Road to three-year-old Frederick son of Alfred Trotter bank accountant.
- Eliza Williams (aged 30 in 1891) – nurse at 9 Brook Street, and head of the household, looking after her 20 year old infirm brother Levi.
- Jane Vaughan (aged 67 in 1891) – retired nurse in Harley Almshouse. Jane was born in Talgarth and

there is a strong possibility that she worked at the Mid-Wales Counties Mental Asylum in the village.
- Anna Brunston (aged 47 in 1901) – nurse at Oakfield to ten-year-old Geffrey son of Thomas Morgan, retired Captain Royal Horse Artillery.

This list provides an indication of the social structure of Hay as much as the number or skill levels of the various individuals who were described as nurses.

In the 1939 census a Miss Edith Gwilliam was termed the matron of the Harley Almshouses. With this title she was possibly a registered nurse employed to support the residents although they were essentially self-caring. Edith was also a member of the Women's Royal Voluntary Service.

In the same census Miss Elizabeth Thomas was described as a retired hospital matron. Born 5 September 1859 she was 80 years old in 1939 and living at 3 Oakland Villas Brecon Road. Where she was matron is unknown but it is possible it was at the Mid Wales Counties Mental Asylum in Talgarth. She was too old to have been employed at the South Wales Sanitorium at Bronllys.

The Hay and Cusop Nursing Association.

The Hay and Cusop Nursing Association was founded in 1903 to celebrate the coronation of King Edward VII.

It relied on donations for income and approached institutions and individuals for a subscription. At its meeting in March 1903 the master of the Workhouse said several outdoor paupers would benefit from the services of the permanent nurse who had been engaged. The workhouse already subscribed three guineas to the Talgarth, Glasbury and Dorstone associations so agreed to do the same to Hay.[8]

During that first year the association managed to raise over £85[9] and employed Nurse Eaton. She attended 109 cases with a total of 1,241 visits. This including 461 in receipt of parish relief. Before the days of the NHS this service was a significant benefit to the community.

Mr H. Studt of the fairground family, who lived in Clyro, was a strong supporter and normally donated the proceeds of the annual Hay May Fair to the association. Between 1903 and 1907 this amounted to nearly £40, greatly assisting them to support those they felt in dire need. In 1908 he deferred his annual contribution to the next year to make a more substantial sum.

The following year when his daughter Louise married the association presented her with a solid silver fruit dish as a token of appreciation for Mr Studt's support.[10] He maintained his contributions, assisted by Mr Tuscon his fellow fairground operator, after the First World War. In 1922 they gave the takings of £21 for one whole evening's rides from the 'Golden Dragon', and again in 1924 when it amounted to over £26.

At the association's annual meeting in 1915, held at Sycamore House, Dr Tom Hincks presided in the absence of Captain E.F. Cockcroft. Their Annual

Report stated that patients from Hay had been sent during the past year to Llandrindod Wells, Hereford and Birmingham Hospitals, and Droitwich Brine Baths.

The appointment of officers for the coming year had been agreed at a meeting of the subscribers on the previous Monday. This took place at Hay Castle, by the kind invitation of Dowager Lady Glanusk. The following appointments were made: President Miss R.M.B. Morgan; vice-president Mrs William Lilwall; joint hon. secs. Mrs Tom Hincks, Mrs T.E. James and Mrs T. Stokoe; hon. treasurer Miss R.M.B. Morgan; executive committee Mrs R.T. Griffiths, Mrs C. Lilwall, Mrs Taylor, Mrs William Lilwall, the Honourable Mabel Bailey, Mrs James Williams and Mrs G. Watkin.[11] Again it can be seen that appointments followed the social structure of the town. The same prominent Hay families were involved in it as in most of the other organisations in the town.

The nursing association was well supported and very active in the inter war period. In 1928 Nurse Lloyd attended 53 cases, with 737 visits including 10 maternity cases. Nurse Spurrier, a part-time nurse who also worked for the county council, attended 18 midwifery cases and 10 maternity cases.[12]

Various social events, plays, recitals and sporting events put on in the town were used as excuses to raise money for the association. Regular support came from the football club and the Hay Drama Group. Mrs Dorothy Nutt wife of the local chemist was secretary in 1940.

The association was still in existence in 1960 when it received a £200 legacy in the will of Mrs Kathleen Booth widow of Major Booth of Cusop.[13]

Matron Alice de Winton. (See Appendix 2 page 211)

An interesting report appeared in The Brecon County Times 5 November 1914.

'Mrs Richard de Winton, wife of Major de Winton, who is now at the front, left Laurel Cottage, Hay, on Tuesday, to take up the appointment of superintendent nurse on a Red Cross hospital train with our Expeditionary Force in France. The train is equipped with 500 beds and Mrs de Winton will have some 30 nurses under her. She has had experience of this work in South Africa.'

Alice was not a native of Hay, in fact she did not live here. Her husband was Major Richard Stratton de Winton. They lived in Cornwall, but Richard's sister Violet May de Winton lived at Laurel Cottage in Church Street.

Alice had trained as a nurse and volunteered for service in South Africa during the Boer War. At the end of it in 1902 she and Richard married.

At the beginning of the First World War Richard went straight to France. As a married woman Alice was ineligible to join the Queen Marys Imperial Nursing Service, despite her Boer War experience. Instead she volunteered for the Red Cross, and used her sister in laws cottage as a staging post on her journey to France.

Matrons did not work on the trains, and in early December Alice was posted to Lady Hadfield's Anglo-American Hospital, Wimereux. By March she was matron of No.2 British Red Cross Hospital, Rouen. This could have included continuing responsibility for the Red Cross ambulance train.

After two years Alice returned to Britain and became matron of an officer's convalescent hospital in Yorkshire. We have no knowledge if she ever returned to Hay.

Voluntary Aid Detachments (V.A.D.'s).

During the Great War the Red Cross set up Voluntary Aid Detachment units to train unqualified men to assist the qualified nursing staff in caring for the troops. Originally only men were recruited with a view that they could serve abroad while women could not.

Rapidly the contingencies of war meant that this outdated view was revised and women were recruited, serving both at home and abroad. The individual members of the detachments quickly becoming known as V.A.D.'s.

The 12th (Hay) Brecknock Voluntary Aid Detachment, British Red Cross, was run by Miss Anna Elizabeth Tunnard-Moore of Cusop.

Dr Valentine Rees of Brecon held an examination of some members on Tuesday 22 February 1916 in the Parish Hall. The results were:

- Five gained their Red Cross Proficiency Badges, - Miss Rosa M.B. Morgan, Miss Rose Byron, Miss Agnes Maddy, Miss Eva Baker, and Miss Elizabeth P. Maddy.
- Two passed their First Aid Re-examination - Miss Alice Pritchard and Miss Ivy Weale.
- Four passed in home nursing - Miss Dorothy Pritchard, Miss Muriel Marwood, Miss Mabel Manning, and Miss Rosalie Grant.

Dr Rees expressed himself as very satisfied with the keenness displayed by the Hay V.A.D. members. He said he knew they must all have felt they owed a deep debt of gratitude to Dr Tom Hincks for the very excellent lectures he must have given them that winter. Dr Rees also alluded to the enthusiastic labours of the commandant, Miss Tunnard-Moore, and congratulated her upon the success of the detachment.[14]

In November 1916 the following Hay nurses had taken up V.A.D. duties.[15]

Miss Eva Baker and Miss Agnes Maddy.

Eva of Oxford Road and Agnes of the Bull Ring worked at Penoyre Red Cross Hospital, Brecon, in May 1916 before going on to the Welsh Hospital, Netley, Hants on 1 November 1916. They were employed as Nurse Probationers Hospital Duties on ward and nursing duties at £20 p.a. Agnes left soon after arriving on 1 February 1917 but Eva remained until 1 November 1918.

Miss Gladys Lilwall.

Gladys of Glanwyn worked as an 'S.G.' Probationer from 29 November 1916 until 7 January 1918 at St John's Hospital, Gloucester Road, Cheltenham Military Hospital.

Miss Alice Wellings.

Alice of Wye Temperance Hotel 10 Castle Street had a more exciting time. Again she was employed as a Nursing Probationer on £20 p.a. From 21 May 1915 to 4 April 1919 she was based at the 5th Southern General Hospital, Portsmouth. During that time she was transferred overseas to Malta from 29 November 1916 to 24 October 1917, first to St. Andrews Hospital, then onto Imtarfa Hospital, before returning to Portsmouth.[16]

Large country houses were requestioned during the First World War as convalescent hospitals. The nearest Red Cross Convalescent Hospitals to Hay were at Brecon and Llyswen, and there was another at Sarnesfield Court in Herefordshire.

Hay Castle mansion was too small but to do her bit for the war Lady Glanusk hosted a number of visits by patients from these hospitals.[17] She also hosted at least one visit by the Red Cross in 1916.[18]

Post War Nursing.

Details of nursing services for Hay and District after the war are sparse. Nurse Lloyd worked on the district, possibly in a private role, during the 1920's and

30's. She attended Katherine Armstrong, the wife of the notorious Hay solicitor Herbert Rowse Armstrong, before she died in 1921.[19]

After the Second World War 'a jolly District Nurse' Jessie Davies travelled around the district by motorbike. She was born at Wye View in Glasbury and died c1974.[20]

Midwifery.

Charles Dickens portrayal of Victorian midwives as gin sodden old gossips is unfair. Certainly they were likely to be mature ladies, but they were respected members of the local population called upon when the need arose. There is limited evidence of any degree of formal training and most would have gained practical experience over the years assisting others.

> **FOUR AT A BIRTH.**
> The Rev. James Paton, curate in charge of the parish of Cusop, Hay, Herefordshire, writes :— "It may interest some of your readers to know that the above rather unusual incident occurred in my parish on the 6th inst., two of the children being born alive. They, with the mother, are doing wonderfully well." Mr. Paton further asserts that the father, a toll-keeper in poor circumstances, and who has already four children to provide for, "though naturally a little confused, seems grateful."

The earliest local record of midwifery is when the bishop of Hereford cathedral licensed two midwifes from Clifford in 1757, Ann Hergest on the

26 March and Katherine Evans on the 13 April.[21] No similar register has been found for Breconshire.

By the 19th century most towns and villages appear to have a formally appointed midwife. Sarah Vaughan was listed in the 1871 census as a midwife in the village of Llandieu.

There is a report in the Lancet and B.M.J. of a midwife in Hay, Mary Price, being taken to court in 1899. Margaret Price died due to loss of blood after Mary had refused to call a doctor or surgeon to assist when the patient collapsed after giving birth. It was alleged that Mary was 'much under the influence of drink', and at the Brecon and Radnor Assize she was sentenced to three years penal servitude.[22]

Following the Midwives Act of 1902 Brecon County Council set up a Health Committee. Dr T.S.H. Hincks was a member. The importance of midwifery services led the county council to approach the Urban District Council in 1908 to seek nominations for a £10 scholarship for midwifery training. The council agreed to advertise the opportunity as well as approach the Hay and Cusop Nursing Association.[23]

In 1914 there was no midwife in Hay and a joint appointment was proposed, to include the medical treatment of schoolchildren and public health work. The council baulked at the salary of £10 p.a. which they viewed to be too much.

This was overcome in September of that year when Miss Banks was appointed to cover the county. Although resident in Talgarth she was also Assistant Sanitary Inspector in Hay, thereby enabling the council to obtain a recharge of £5 from the treasury.

Dr Tom Hincks gave an insight into midwifery locally in 1929 in an article in the B.M.J. In his view things had improved a great deal in the previous 15 years but there was still no maternity nurse in the Herefordshire part of his practice. In Radnorshire a nurse had been appointed in every district, under the supervision of a district nursing association. Each was subsidised at a cost of £50 p.a. paid for by the county council.

He reported prejudice still existed against the nurses for washing the mother and changing the soiled garments and bedlinen after delivery. Apparently this was due to concerns that the mother might catch a chill, but was being gradually overcome.

He also explained that folklore customs still persisted. If the baby had been delivered by the time he arrived frequently he found that the chord was tied by a piece of string to the mothers leg. Her fingers may also have a piece of wool wound around them to prevent haemorrhaging.[24]

Pharmacy services.

Travelling quacks were a feature of rural life until well into the 19th century, and regularly appeared at the spring and autumn Hiring Fairs in Hay.

They were entirely different from the mendicants, the wandering charmers such as the Dyn Hysbys or cunning men who had a strong tradition in early Welsh medicine. These men developed considerable skills, and herbs assumed increasing importance in their healing repertoire.

Over time this meant that the role of the mendicant evolved into that of the apothecary. Initially they stored herbs and spices, as well as wine to mix them with, and all of which were available to buy. It was only a matter of time before they started creating and selling their own medicines, and the role of the apothecary was born.

They were formally recognised by a Royal Charter in 1617 and by around 1650 apothecaries had become established in most towns.

We know there were a number of apothecaries in Hay. The parish records for April 1785 show that the Overseers was instructed to approach them to find the one who would give the most advantageous terms for attending the poor for the following year.

Apothecaries stock in Wales were not so different from that seen in the capital They sold a wide variety of pills and potions, oils and powders. London dealers often had Welsh agents. Their work was codified by the Apothecaries Act of 1815, and this allowed them to give medical advice as well as prescribe medicines.

Dr Gwynne James of Kington (died 18 June 1801) had an extensive joint practice with his father, and was respected enough to be consulted by others. In his journal of 1770-75 he recorded the use of his own preparations, no doubt evolved over many years, as well as those from the London Pharmacopoeia.

In addition he would have had a number of propriety medicines available which were in general use.

- Scott's Pills were a universal panacea. These were used by the 1806 Lewis and Clark Expedition in America to treat three men. They appear to have been used as a cathartic and only one patient benefited following the administration of 12 pills. In the 19th century they were used for constipation and gastric or bilious complaints.
- Bracken Pills were given for worms.
- Holloways Ointment for ulcerations and sores, ringworm and erysipelas (a skin infection).
- Dovers Powder (Pulv. Ipecach Co) was a painkiller reputedly evolved by a pirate, but in practice developed by Dr Thomas Dover. It was reportedly in use in Trinidad by the Royal Navy as early as 1818, and only removed from the list of approved medicines in the U.K. in the 1960's.
- Daffys Elixir was developed by the Rev. Thomas Daffy in 1647, and knowledge of it passed down through his family. It was a herbal mixture using rhubarb, fennel seeds, aniseed, parsley, raisins, saffron, senna and Spanish liquorice amongst other ingredients, dissolved in brandy. It was primarily a laxative but had a reputation as a 'cure all' for almost anything, or measure of last resort![25]

As the apothecaries skills in understanding the action of medicines on the body developed a new profession, that of pharmacist, was established in 1841. Professional standards were set and they lobbied very hard to ensure drugs were only sold by those qualified to do so. It was largely due to their efforts that restrictions on the way arsenic was sold were introduced.

In Hay there have been a number of chemist/pharmacy stores.

HOOPER, Thomas.

In 1841 a 35-year-old druggist Thomas Hooper was living in Castle Street. He would have sold the gallon stone jar (contents unknown) marked T. Hooper Chemist Hay, and found relatively recently at Hill Farm, Llanigon. The London Gazette reported Thomas was declared bankrupt 12 August 1842.[26]

STOKOE, Thomas J.

Thomas Stokoe became a very prominent member of the Hay community. He was born near Gateshead in 1838, and first appeared in Hay in 1861 as a shop assistant to Benjamin Hadley who ran a chemist shop. Three years later Thomas had qualified in Edinburgh as a veterinary surgeon but he found veterinary work too physically demanding. Instead he became the proprietor of Benjamin's shop at 12 High Town where he had worked when he first arrived.

Benjamin retired to run his father's farm, but he and Thomas went into partnership in 1870 to open a grocers, off licence and druggists in Castle Street. George Sampson Valentine Wills was engaged to manage it.

George was born in Roade, Northamptonshire, and initially worked for a local healer 'Doctor' Cashmere. This inspired him to become a pharmacist. From 1866 he was apprenticed to a couple of local pharmacists before moved to Hay as manager.

While in Hay George continued studying for his pharmacy qualification and took his preliminary examination in Hereford. He also met Miss Goode, a resident of Hay, during his stay. After two years he moved on to Barrow-in-Furness but returned to Hay 30 September 1874 to marry Miss Goode. George later found teaching his vocation and opened his very successful Westminster College of Chemistry and Pharmacy in London. Among his 4,000 or more pharmacy students was a Mr Jones who set up practice in Erwood near Brecon.

In addition to the grocers, druggists and off license shop in Castle Street, Thomas went on to own the Wine Vaults at 10 Castle Street and several pubs. After 1891 his acquisitions also included the Crown Hotel in Broad Street, run by the efficient Miss Kisbey.

Thomas retained an interest in veterinary work, especially horses, but it was his Stokoes Sheep Dip that was his greatest achievement. It was a great commercial success both in the UK and in Australia. A five-gallon earthenware bottle exists with his name on it but unfortunately there is no mention of whether its contents were sheep dip.

DAVIS, John Lutwyche.

John was born in 1825 in Hay. In the 1891 census he was described as a chemist living at 22 Broad Street. It is known he established the present pharmacy at 7 High Town in the 1850's, and he was succeeded by his son Fred.

DAVIS, Fred.

Fred was born in 1860 and lived at Clifton House 1 Belmont Road two doors up from Dr Tom Hincks. Fred achieved notoriety as the instigator of the investigation that led to Herbert Rowse Armstrong being hung for the murder of his wife Katherine in the famous Hay murder trial of 1922.[27]

Armstrong was the solicitor who always acted for Fred, but he assisted a chemists assistant Mr Esdras Sant to establish a drug shop in Hay.

Esdras worked for Thomas Stokoe but when Thomas retired Esdras lost his job. He asked Armstrong for advice. Based on this he opened Sants Drug Store, selling everything Fred sold except registered drugs. As a result Esdras became quite successful.

Fred was aggrieved at the help Armstrong had given Esdras to set up in competition to him. He had expected to operate a monopoly on Stokoe's retirement. This is thought to be why he acted as he did against Armstrong. After the trial Fred was ostracised and left Hay in 1924.

Fred, or his assistant, had sold the white arsenic to Armstrong in the first place. This contravened the law requiring arsenic to be coloured before sale. It is perhaps poetic justice that sometime after he left Hay Fred was prosecuted by the Pharmaceutical Council for selling unadulterated white arsenic.

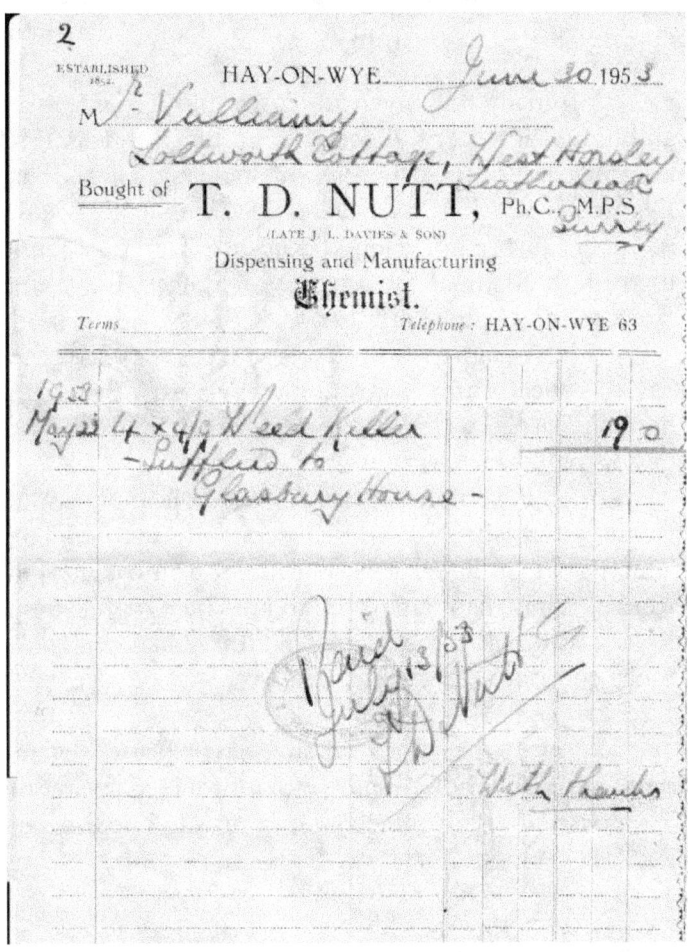

NUTT, Thomas Dixon.

When Fred Davis left Hay his chemists shop was purchased by pharmacist Thomas Dixon Nutt

M.P.S. Ph.C.. He had been born in Goole Yorkshire and served his apprenticeship at J.G. Twiggs a chemist at Withenshaw, going on to marry Twiggs daughter Dorothy.

Initially they lived in Cusop but Thomas was ambitious and very successful in his business. He became chair of the Chamber of Trade and Hay Urban District Council.[28] They were also both enthusiastic members of the golf club. Thomas had a house built high on the bank at the junction of Forrest Road and Brecon Road in the early 1930's.

His daughter Jeanne would cross the road each day to collect water from the nearby Swan Well. This highly regarded water source was for use in the house rather than the pharmacy.

Jeanne entered the Foreign Office and went to Russia. Here she met and subsequently married Ian, later Sir Ian, Sutherland who become an ambassador in Russia. They had an exciting life, being posted in Russia, Cuba and the United States at key events in those countries, and world, history.[29]

Over the years there have been several buildings throughout the town that provided shelter or care for ill or disadvantaged inhabitants in one form or another.

Union Workhouse.

Although workhouses were not hospitals or care homes as we understand them today, they were important welfare centres.

Until relatively recently there was no national system of support for the poor. For centuries parishes were responsible for providing food, accommodation, and care for the unemployed, homeless, sick and elderly. Standards varied widely. The Poor Law Amendment Act 1834 was introduced to establish a national system and standard for the provision of Poor Relief. This included the building of workhouses.

Four workhouses were built in Breconshire. The Hay Poor Law Union covering the eastern boundary of Breconshire, southern Radnorshire and Western Herefordshire. It was amongst the first wave and was established on the 26 September 1836. It covered the following 25 parishes in the three counties, with a combined population of 11,403 in 1831.

- Breconshire – Aberllynfy, Bonllys, Glynfach, Capel-y-fin, Hay, Llaneilieu, Llanigan, Llyswen, Pipton, Talgarth (including Borough, Forest, Trefecca, Pwll-y-wrach, Tregoyd, and Velindre).
- Radnorshire – Bettws Clyro, Boughrood, Bryngwn, Clyro, Glasbury, Llanbedr-Painscastle, Llandeilo Graban, Llanstephan, Llowes.
- Herefordshire – Bredwardine, Cusop, Clifford, Dorstone, Whitney.[30]

The workhouse was built in 1837, opposite St Mary's Church, and cost £3,200. Originally only meant to house 15 inmates it had extensive additions and alterations in subsequent years to enlarge it and bring it up to the required standard.

The design was a typical cruciform shape with a central administrative core and four radiating arms, one each for males, females, infirm and able-bodied. The whole was bounded by railings and iron gates.[31]

To administer the workhouse, and care for the poor, a Board of Guardians was set up. This consisted of 27 local ratepayers, one from each parish and two each from Hay and Pwll-y-wrach. The Guardians appointed a master and matron to run it, and Mr Henry Proctor as the appointed surgeon with the Rev. Allen of Hay to care for their spiritual needs.

Shortly after the workhouse opened it was decided that the arm of the building used for the infirmary was not adequate and it needed its own hospital. A number of advertisements appeared on 10 September 1846 inviting tenders to erect a new building.[32]

The hospital was known as Union House and evolved into a kind of general medical centre with its own ward. As well as treating patients from the workhouse it cared for those in the general population who could not afford to pay for private care.

It appears users of the hospital were not automatically given medical care. When Mrs Greenway gave birth in 1868 her child died. Dr Bogle laid a complaint against the Relieving Officer, William Powell, because he did not call for Dr Bogle to attend. The newspaper report noted that 'neither the man nor wife had provided a medical man'. Presumably this meant they were too poor to pay for one. The Relieving Officer gave his reasons for not calling for medical assistance to the Guardians, and again this might have been finance based. He was exonerated from blame.[33]

Another patient who was not an inmate of the workhouse was pig farmer Jeremiah Price. He lived with his daughter and granddaughter in Boughrood. Jeremiah became ill in 1877 and he was admitted to the hospital. When he died he was taken back to Boughrood by train to be buried.

Nurses appointed to the workhouse infirmary would have worked at Union House. They included Ann Shatton in 1851, Elizabeth Smith in 1861, Eliza Price in 1871, Mary Scott in 1881, Annie Worth in 1891. Sarah Meecham in 1901 and Catherine Edith Banks in 1911.

Once the workhouse buildings were enlarged the number of inmates increased from the original 15 to around 50, although it did vary. The 1861 census listed 54 inmates with an equal number of males and females, and approximately one third of these were young children. Families were split up on entry which was a further sign of degradation.

Despite the large catchment area less than six inmates came from a greater distance than ten miles from Hay. They were from Ross, Llandrindod, Llandeilo, and one female who came originally from London.

Conditions were spartan and bleak, with poor food and a large number of strict rules. All able-bodied men were required to work, breaking stones for road making in the cellar or picking oakum, while women had to attend to washing and cleaning.

Oakham picking, to make caulk for ships, was used to take up any 'spare' time of both men and women. This involved unpicking tarred hemp cables that were too rotten to use. A spike was used to push into the ropes but due to the tar it was very difficult and hard on the fingers and hands. Everyone hated it.

However hard life was at the workhouse there were attempts to provide some light relief. In July 1906 Mr and Mrs Robert Griffiths of Trewern, Cusop, hosted an afternoon outing for the inmates. After being shown round the pretty garden tea was served to everyone. The children in particular enjoyed themselves 'hay making'.[34]

The Poor Law Act was amended in 1837 to require parishes to provide a meal and one night's shelter to anyone passing in 'sudden or urgent necessity' in return for performing a simple task. Essentially this was provision for vagrants known as casual poor or 'casuals'.

Initially workhouses put them in the infirmary as they often carried infectious disease but after a time purpose-built single-story buildings were used. Conditions here were even worse that in the workhouse to further discourage anyone 'taking to the road'.

At Hay a small room by the main gates was reserved for them. Prior to that they were placed wherever there was space.

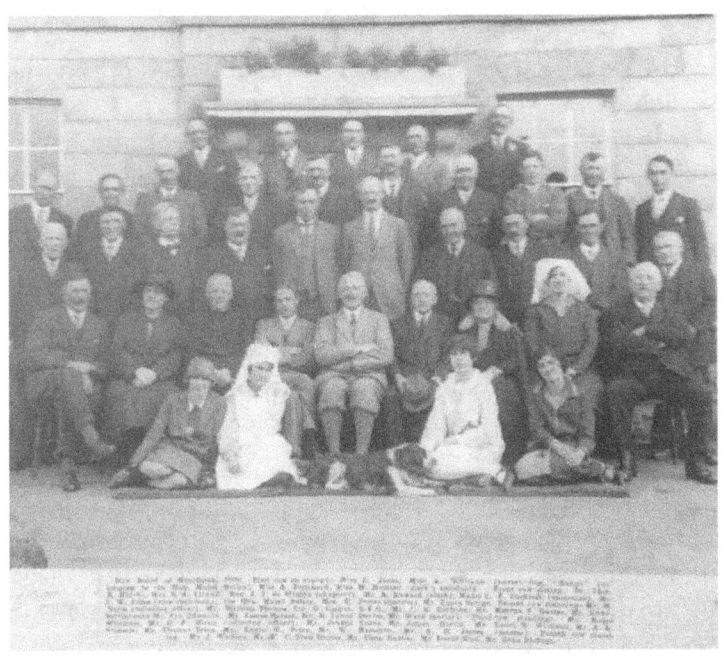

Hay Board of Guardians (early 1920's?). Dr Tom Hincks was medical officer (second row extreme left). In addition to Nurse Miss A. Williams (front row). Union House also had a matron Mrs Edna E.G. James (second row).[35]

The Visiting Committee found on an inspection of the 'tramp wards' that three vagrants were sometimes placed in a bathroom, and two or three 'were put together' on other wards.[36] This was unsatisfactory and later a reduced number of places were filled on a first come first accommodated basis. Excess applicants were simply turned away.

That this service fulfilled a need is illustrated by the minutes of the Local Board meeting on 11 September 1902. At it the master reported that 51 vagrants had 'been relieved' through the workhouse in the past fortnight. This was an increase of seven compared to the same period the previous year.[37]

Despite the degradation and poor conditions workhouse inmates had at least some form of food, and shelter at night. This gave those who had fallen on hard times a basic form of welfare, and if they became ill they would get a bed in the infirmary and the chance to see the workhouse doctor.

Hospitals.

Because of the facilities at Union House on the workhouse site Hay never had a dedicated cottage hospital. This was despite Mr H. Studt of the fairground family voicing his support for one saying he would support both the building and the ongoing running costs.[38]

This was typical of the charitable work done in Hay by Mr Studt, particularly for the Nursing Association. In acknowledgement of this in 1935 he was presented with an illuminated address by the Hay Urban District Council.[39]

The town also made use of the workhouse mortuary. As there was no official mortuary vehicle the horse bus normally used to ferry passengers from the railway station into town was used. This meant the transportation of any infected deceased became an issue. In 1876 the clerk to the Local Board felt it necessary to write to the owners to advise them that:

> *'in any future cases in which they may convey any deceased person who died from any infectious or contagious disease ... the Board will institute proceedings unless they immediately provide the disinfection of such conveyance.'*[40]

Fairs notes that on one occasion there was a delay in transporting a body. To hasten events the doctor concerned dressed the deceased in outdoor clothes, sat him in the front seat of his car and ferried him to the mortuary, without anyone having cause to make comment.

Isolation Hospital (also known as the Fever Hospital).

By virtue of its position off the normal trade routes Hay did not suffer greatly from some of the major epidemics affecting other towns. However like most small towns it had outbreaks of infectious diseases. Smallpox, measles, and scarlet fever occurred regularly. These were attributed to local vagrants calling at the workhouse, and with some justification.

The outbreaks were a constant possibility, and a worry to the local authorities. They led to the schools being closed on numerous occasions. Particularly bad years were 1895/6 when they were shut from 25 June to 7 October due to scarlet fever, and then 1 January to 2 March due to measles.

These outbreaks led to protracted standoffs between the Local Board and the Guardians of Hay Union. In addition to the arrival of vagrants who sought accommodation overnight, the Local Board complained about the general filth and overcrowding at the workhouse. They felt this was a contributory factor to the outbreak of scarlet fever in 1879-80. It was at times like these that the lack of an isolation hospital was noted.

The Isolation Hospital Acts of 1893 and 1901 empowered County Councils to take responsibility for scarlet fever, diphtheria and similar notifiable infectious diseases. Costs, as always, were a major disincentive for councils and hence they were slow to take any action. In Hay a suggestion that Gypsy Castle Cottage be acquired for isolation purposes came to nought.

After the report of a case of smallpox at Tunk's Common Lodging House at 11 Chancery Lane in 1893 it was decided to try and create a temporary isolation hospital in a small cottage, Cardigan Hall. This occupied an isolated position near the top of Common Lane on the hill above the cemetery.

In the event this was not followed up and the smallpox case was successfully isolated at the lodging house. Three vagrants who had been in contact were successfully housed in the isolation ward of Union House.

The subject was briefly discussed again in 1894 but no action was taken. In 1902 an outbreak of scarlet fever in Newport Street and Heol y Dwr led to the renting of a cottage in Oxford Road.

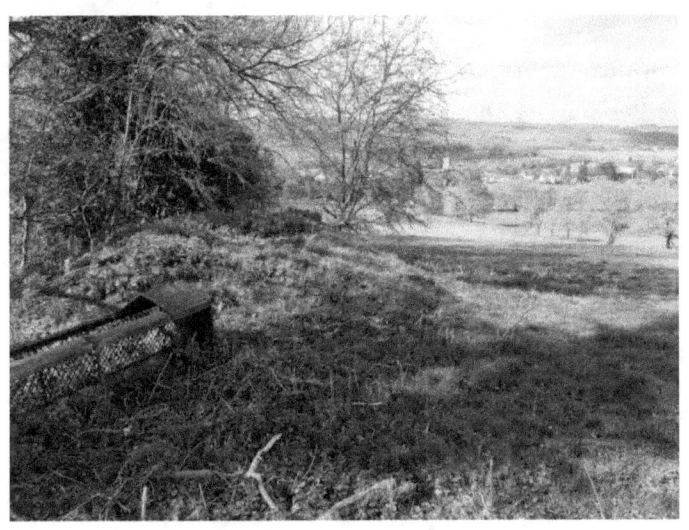

The site of Cardigan Hall, now a mound of rubble.

That same year a tramp with smallpox was placed in a tent at Cardigan Hall.[41] It was later reported at a Hay Urban District Council meeting that the use of tents allowed very little space for treatment. It had also cost £70 with further costs for a second case. Members were encouraged to try again to get the three rural districts and Hay Urban District Council to agree to combine to provide an isolation hospital.

A committee was set up to make enquiries regarding the costs and suitability of a site.[42] They noted that the previous year the papers had reported that following a tender Messrs Davies and Maltby of Hereford had been placed first for their designs and plans for an isolation hospital.[43] Previously they had designed the hospital at Leominster.[44]

As usual nothing much appears to have happened for a number of years. Eventually on the 10 January 1910 the council considered the offers of land for the hospital by Viscount Hereford and Lord Glanusk. After inspecting a site in Gypsy Castle Lane attached to the workhouse the council resolved to accept Lord Glanusk's offer of Gypsy Castle Cottage in Warren Lane, the first house visible from the bend at the railway abutments.

There was further delay until they met again on 7 August 1910 following another epidemic of scarlet fever. This time they acted. A site was chosen and secured, a committee formed and a fund set up. The Rev. G. Leigh Spencer of The Priory Clifford was made the treasurer.

By early 1911 the money was secured from Hay and the surrounding parishes from voluntary contributions.

	£	s	d
Hay Town	106	7	6
Clifford	74	4	4
Clyro	50	15	6
Cusop	44	10	6
Tregoyd/Velindre	36	6	0
Glasbury	29	19	0
Llanigan	8	11	6
Dorstone	4	4	0
Llowes	1	0	0
Outside subscribers	31	3	0
Entertainments	37	1	8
Bank interest	3	7	0
Total	427	10	0

The hospital cost £353 10s 5 to erect. It consisted of a simple wooden building with corrugated iron cladding, similar to many around the country. Two bungalows were also built on site for staff. An additional £70 covered the cost of furniture and equipment which was purchased from the Hay Urban District Council. Printing and postage to set the hospital up came to £4.

A letter in the Hereford Journal shows the first chairman was Mr R.C. Devereux. Predictably Dr Hinks was appointed as Inspector of the Isolation Hospital at £3. 3s. 0d. pa and £1. 1s. 0d. attendance fee. Any woman employed to nurse one case was to be given 10s a week, 20s. for two cases and 25s. for additional cases. They also had to look after the premises.

Patients from Bredwardine, Painscastle and Hay were to be admitted at £1. 1s. 0d. a case plus £1. 1s. 0d. and expenses for Dr Hincks. There was space for six adults or 15 children.

By November 1913 there were six cases of scarlet fever from outside the district admitted. Interestingly no beds appear to have been procured initially so that when the six patients were admitted Dr Hincks had to find beds for them.

Money was always an issue. In 1913 a closed conveyance to be used as an ambulance for the hospital was lent by Mr Thomas Lloyd proprietor of the Rhydspence Inn. In January 1914 he reclaimed his waggon because the council was not prepared to pay for it.

The hospital was only used intermittently. During the summer of 1917 female undergraduates from Oxford and Cambridge undertook farm work to support the war effort. Seven ladies from Girton College Cambridge came to work at Clyro and were billeted at the hospital. They left after two months work. [45]

In 1918 Major Walford, the sanitary specialist based in Cardiff, enquired if there were any local arrangements for military cases to be admitted. The council replied that they could take up to eight cases at the normal terms of £1. 1s. 0d for a doctor with additional expenses for nursing, maintenance, etc. at cost.

After the war, on 7 July 1919, the council agreed that the fee for cases admitted from outside the district should increase from £1. 1s. 0d. to £2. 2s. 0d.

It is not known how busy the hospital was but in its latter days it was reserved exclusively for youngsters with infectious diseases.

The hospital closed in 1948 at the inception of the NHS and the site was then converted into a farm. On 24 January 1950 the executors of Lord Glanusk formally transferred the site, buildings and 0.997 acres of land to the Urban District Council for £95. [46]

Mid -Wales Counties Mental Asylum.

There was mention of a Talgarth Asylum in 1872 (see Dr Coulson) but no record of it has been found. The Brecon and Radnor Joint Lunatic Asylum at Talgarth cost £126,000 to build and was opened in 1903 by Lord Glanusk. By 1914 it was one of a network of 102 across England and Wales.

The asylum was a major employer in the area. A number of people from Hay worked there, and it also had a few patients from the town.

Like other such institutions it was designed to be self-sufficient. As well as its own farm it had independent utilities, such as water, electricity, heating and sewerage systems.

Although originally set up only for patients from Brecon and Radnor, after the First World War it started to accepted patients from Montgomeryshire as well. This led to its renaming as the Mid-Wales Counties Mental Asylum. The Mid and West Wales College of Nursing and Midwifery was set up there.

During the Second World War the asylum opened a military section, and it is rumoured that Rudolph Hess, the Nazi leader, stayed there one night when passing through. Hay cemetery has a small number of Commonwealth War Graves Commission headstones to foreign soldiers who ended their days at Talgarth. After the war it reverted to civilian use.

Like all such institutions once admitted many patients became institutionalised and fewer than half were ever discharged. In the 1980's the asylum went into decline with the introduction of the Care in the Community initiative. It finally closed in 1999 and the site is now derelict.

South Wales Sanitorium, Bronllys.

As a lasting memorial to King Edward VII, in 1910 Wales decided that it would create a campaign for the eradication of tuberculosis. Accordingly on the 17 May 1912 the King Edward VII Welsh National

Memorial Association was established by Royal Charter.

Exactly one year later Pontywal House and its grounds at Bronllys, seven miles from Hay, was acquired, as well as 373 extra acres of land. The county surveyor Mr Edwards designed the South Wales Sanitorium tuberculosis hospital, and it was opened by King George V and Queen Mary in 1920.

Facilities were created to treat 256 adults and 48 boys. Presumably girls did not get TB! With the post war decline in tuberculosis the sanitorium finally closed in 1999.

The old sanitorium was then renamed Bronllys Hospital. It retains one ward run by GP's as well as a wide range of outpatient services.

The site is currently being developed as a Well Being Park.

Notes.
[1] *Hereford Times* (6 October 1838).
[2] *Hereford Times* (24 November 1848).
[3] *Hereford Journal* (25 November 1848).
[4] *Brecon County Times* (26 June 1919).
[5] *Haywire* 66.
[6] *Staffordshire Sentinel* (11 December 1993).
[7] Bennett, David. (2015) *Local History in the Pubs and Inns of Hay*. Lulu.
[8] *Brecon County Times* (27 March 1903).
[9] *Brecon County Times* (1 April 1904).
[10] *Brecon County Times* (16 April 1909).
[11] *Hereford Times* (April 1915).
[12] *Brecon County Times* (3 May 1928).
[13] *Birmingham Daily Post* (20 August 1960).
[14] *Brecon County Times* (March 1916).
[15] *Hereford Times* (30 November 1916).
[16] Red Cross. https://vad.redcross.org.uk.
[17] *Brecon County Times* (January 1916).
[18] *Brecon County Times* (17 August 1916).
[19] *Leeds Mercury* (26 January 1922).
[20] *Haywire* 61.
[21] Moir, L.A., Schoolmasters and surgeons licensed by the Bishop of Hereford and schoolmasters licensed by the Dean and Chapter of Hereford, 1683-1835. *Transactions of the Woolhope Club* (1952) 135-139.
[22] *Shepton Mallet Journal* (17 November 1899).
[23] *Radnor Express* (16 July 1908).
[24] Hincks, T.E., British Medical Association, *B.M.J.* (24 August 1929) 346.
[25] *Hereford Times* (19 September 1846).
[26] *Liverpool Standard and General Commercial Advertiser* (12.08.1842).
[27] Beales, Martin, *The Hay Poisoner,* Robert Hale (1995).
[28] Hull Daily Mail (26 April 1940).
[29] Sutherland, Jeanne, *From Moscow to Cuba and Beyond. A Diplomatic Memoir of the Cold War.* Radcliff Press (London, 2010).

[30] *Hereford Journal* (15 November 1862).
[31] Fairs Geoffrey, *A History of the Hay*, Phillimore (Chichester, 1974).
[32] *Hereford Times* (19 September 1846).
[33] *Brecon County Times* (22 August 1868).
[34] *Cusop Church magazine*, September 1906.
[35] Photograph courtesy of E.&T. Pugh.
[36] *Brecon County Times* (17 April 1896).
[37] *Brecon County Times* (12 September 1902).
[38] *Brecon and Radnor Express & Carmarthenshire Times* (28 May 1908).
[39] *Western Mail* (14 December 1935).
[40] Fairs, Geoffrey. (1972) *The History of Hay*, Chichester, Phillimore.
[41] Ibid.
[42] *Hereford Journal* (28 March 1903).
[43] *Hereford Journal* (10 May 1902).
[44] *Ross Gazette* (8 May 1902).
[45] *Brecon County Times* (12 July 1917).
[46] Nicholls, A.J., *Historical Directory of Hay on Wye. Rural Parish* (Lulu, 2016).

Chapter 6 – Medical Services

While herbal healers like the descendants of Physicians of Myddfai could do an excellent job for their times, an increased level of skill were required to support the health of the growing population.

Initially apothecaries had fulfilled this role but gradually, as new knowledge and skills developed, the day of the physician had arrived.

Doctors and Surgeons.

Today the terms doctor and surgeon denote medical professionals with different but equal levels of skill. The evolution of the role of the surgeon however was very different from that of the doctor.

From the time of the fall of Rome all education of any sort had been largely in the hands of the church. The word doctor comes from Latin and means 'I teach'. As a result monks were known as doctors because of their teaching role. They were also the people who provided the majority of healthcare. This was at a time when the 'doctor' was not usually called until after the priest had heard the patients, often final, confession.

Later the church decreed that the patients religious welfare took precedence over their physical health. As a consequence it banned any training in medicine. Monks were not allowed to do any surgery. This led to the barbers who attended the tonsures of the monks becoming barber-surgeons.

The decline of monasteries in the Middle Ages meant they became known simply as surgeons. Others with a degree of anatomical knowledge, such as butchers or abattoir workers, also joined their ranks. A similar role developed for the supervision of the health of men in the militia to ensure they were fit to fight.

These were practical men rather than theorists. The word surgery comes from the Greek meaning working with hands, and early surgery was a very rough and ready business. Traditional guidance was 'whatever you do, do it quickly', this in the age of no anaesthetics and with friends holding the patient down on the table.

Physicians and Doctors.

Originally doctors were men who had obtained a degree from a university. These first doctorate degrees covered a wide range of subjects. Each student had to study politics, philosophy and law as well as works of medicine, such as the Greek physician Galen.

Over time the subjects they studied became more specialised so that eventually a doctorate would be obtained in one academic subject. To denote a Doctor of Medicine the term physician was used. This showed that they had a specialist knowledge of physiology, that is, how the body functions.

Doctors could register to practice medicine in one of three ways:

- obtain a license from a bishop in the local diocese.
- graduate from Cambridge or Oxford.
- graduate from one of the Royal Colleges of Medicine.

To do so required effort and money. As a consequence doctors were not only at a higher academic level but they also were of a higher social standing than surgeons. They provided a wider range of healthcare. Doctors directed the work of the less qualified surgeons. As a consequence surgeons were simply known as 'Mr'.

Medical Training.

Early medical books were either translated from the Latin, or written, in English. It was not until 1732 that the first Welsh language medical book was printed. This meant prior to this practitioners who spoke only Welsh were at a serious disadvantage. Even for those with a good knowledge of English there was no medical training centre in Wales.

The first Welsh faculty of medicine was not established in Cardiff until in 1893, but students were still required to go to London to complete their studies. Often those who left to study did not return. They could earn far more money outside the poor rural areas of their homeland.

It was not until 1921 that a complete Medical School was finally opened in Cardiff. This was only due to the generous private sponsorship of Sir William James Thomas and Colonel E.M. Bruce-Vaughan.

Another consequence of the lack of facilities in Wales was that few men bothered to complete all the necessary medical training. None the less they would still call themselves doctor, surgeon, physician, or something similar. In practice until relatively recent times treatment by a skilled partially trained healing practitioner was probably just as effective as many of the early qualified doctors.

The General Medical Council was formed following the Medicines Act of 1858, and it drew up the first register of medical practitioners. This was before the advent of formal medical qualifications, and consequently registrants were elected to the register. Initially a number of healing practitioners who were then practicing in Hay were added, even though they had minimal medical qualifications.

The personal qualities of these men were as important as any medical training. They had to be hardy and practical, forever travelling by horseback on their rounds in all weathers, traversing bogs and streams and climbing steep mountain slopes.

With them they had to carry enough medical supplies to cope with almost any emergency. Roads were poor, and often non-existent in isolated rural homesteads. In difficult conditions the horse might falter requiring the doctor to walk miles up hills and across fells in the rain and snow.

While they maintained their own practices this did not mean they did not cooperate with colleagues, and sometimes employ assistants. Almost certainly they had informal cooperative working arrangements enabling them to support one another when a second opinion was needed, or more specialist help was required.

Medical Practitioners in Hay.

For a small rural market town Hay appears to have had an astonishing number of surgeons, physicians or G.P.'s over the past 250 years. Possibly the large rural hinterland influenced this. On the other hand we do not know how long some of them remained in practice in the town, or whether they worked full or part-time, or came here in semi-retirement.

One factor may have been that there were a relatively low number of patients willing or able to afford their services until the later Victorian period. Perhaps as a consequence many early doctors were part-time farmers or horse breeders. Dr Williams of Talgarth was a noted horse breeder, and with Dr Williams of Brecon and Dr Howells of Talgarth was a frequent exhibitor at county shows.[1]

In 1882 Mr John Edwin Hope a retired grocer of 8 Lion Street wrote a letter to his son Dr James William Hope of Freemantle Australia:[2]

'I don't think either of the doctors in Hay get £300 per year and without private income it is impossible for them to live....'

In 1884 he wrote in a further letter:

'at present I am only just able to drag along from rheumatic pains....I have very little faith in the Hay doctors who have so little practice that they would make a long case of me.'

John Hope's comments are interesting. They conflict with the records that show more than two doctors practicing concurrently in the town throughout much of the 19th century. In 1858 Drs Trumper, Lyde, Proctor and Reece had surgeries in town, and in 1868 we have Bogle, Lyde, Proctor, Smith and Trumper.

However in 1882, at the time of John Hoper's letter, only Dr E.A. Appleby and Dr Thomas S.H. Hincks were in practice. Both were newcomers to the town. Dr Trumper was still living in Brook Street. He had retired from practice although he lived for another 31 years.

It could be that an old superstition in the area might have played a part in their level of income. It was said that in Hay it was unlucky to pay a doctor's bill in full. If you did it was thought that you were shortly going to need further medical assistance. It was best to withhold a small amount. On the other hand perhaps this was just an excuse not to pay the bill in full.

Not everyone was in favour of their services of course. William Beevan of Llanthomas died in 1879 at the age of 105 years claiming to have never needing the services of a doctor. He had a minor ailment when he was 100 and his friends thought it prudent to call a doctor to see him. William felt otherwise and hid in a cupboard until the doctor left.[3]

The earliest local names we have of practitioners of the healing arts in the area are two surgeons licensed by the bishop in Hereford. They were Richard Hantorne of Whitney on 5 October 1683 and John Smith of Clifford on the 20 October 1759.

In Hay a Dr Smith is mentioned in 1727, and Ann Wellington was described as the widow of Edward Wellington, a surgeon (or possibly an apothecary) in 1759. There are no other mentions of any medical man in the town prior to a private Medical Register for Flint published in 1780. This listed three local surgeon-apothecaries, James (J.W.P?) Lyde, John Jones and James Bevan. They were also listed in the Medical Register for the Year 1783. A James Jarvis was later mentioned in a rate book of 1825.

From that date on there are an increasing number of local and national directories (Kellys, Robsons, Slaters, Pigots), as well as official records and census returns, so it is possible to identify more individuals.

ADCOCK, Dr Katherine M.

The 1939 census lists a Miss Adcock at Epyl, Oxford Road and describes her as a part time emergency medical officer. Nothing else is known.

ANDERSON, Dr William Maurice E.D.S.O.

Dr (Bill) Anderson was a G.P. in Hay during the 1960s. Widely respected, he had a good bedside manner and an excellent medical reputation. Local gossip was that he had been the doctor with the first party of paratroopers over Pegasus Bridge on D Day.

This story may have arisen because Lieutenant-Colonel Maurice Anderson 63162 D.S.O. commanded the 195th (Airlanding) Field Ambulance, a Royal Army Medical Corps (R.A.M.C.) unit in the British 6th Airborne Division.

His unit was involved on D Day June 1944, the Allied Invasion of Normandy. They landed at 21.00 on the 6 June from Horsa and Hamilcar gliders at Ranville near the Pegasus and Horsa bridges. Quickly establishing themselves and opening a main dressing station they started treating patients almost immediately. The ten doctors worked in two teams, and by midnight on the 7 June had performed 23 operations. On each of the two succeeding days they performed 11 more operations, often while under sustained mortar fire.

Dr Anderson was badly injured in 1944 while working at a First Aid Post. Despite his injuries, and a number of his patients getting killed, he organised an evacuation to the Main Dressing Station where he then had his wounds dressed.

Two stories about his time in Hay were published in HayWire, the infamous Hay newsletter, (no.77 September 1997, p.5).

These stories may have a touch of exaggeration but show something of Dr Anderson's convivial character, and his reputed love of Scotland's national drink. They are told in a manner that illustrate his patients love and affection for their highly respected local G.P.

Dr Anderson's Wee Dram by Tyke Hyett.
"Did you know Dr Anderson?? No! An'well, anyway, we had a bloke round yer, Scotch bloke, doctor he was. H-h-h-e-i-i! he was a chap who loiked a 'nip'! One day, when he was off-duty - thank God! - and Hay didn't have a lot of traffic, this'd be 1961, the doctor went to a party at "Penywrlodd", Llanigon. And he knocked back the whisky. He managed to drive back to Hay alright, and he parked his car opposite his surgery at Compton House in Hightown. But, when he opened his car door, the cold air must've got him, because he fell out of the car! Drunk as a lord, he crawled across the road on his hands and knees! (Laughter) ... Hell, he was a mon for his wee dram."

Tot From A Scot.
I remember being in Hay in 1973 when a dog bit me and I had to go to the local surgery for a few stitches. A silver-haired doctor attended me; I think he was a Scotsman. Half-way through the stitching he suddenly stopped and took a whisky flask from his pocket and had a drink. He then offered the flask to me which I gratefully accepted, drinking a greedy draught, hoping to numb the pain. "Oh I see you're a whisky man," he said, winking. "Let's do these other two stitches and we'll have a tot of the real McCoy." ... To cut a long story short, we had a two-hour conversation while drinking his 'best malt'. We were the only people in the building. He entertained me with war stories and cheered me up no end.
(Ed. This may have been the late Dr Anderson).

Dr Anderson wrote to the B.M.J. on a couple of occasions. In 1963[4] he commented on a hypothesis put forward on why Queen Ann had so many miscarriages in her 17 pregnancies. Then in 1966[5] he complained about proposed new remuneration arrangements that might disadvantage G.P.'s compared to hospital consultants.

Dr Bill Anderson died in 1986 aged 78.

APPLEBY, Dr Edward.

Dr Appleby was born in Ireland. It is not known where he qualified but by 1881 he was working at Pemberton House Surgery in the Bull Ring. He succeeded Dr Clouston who had retired and moved to London the previous year.

He was the Medical Officer to the Local Board from 1880-6 but by 1891 he had left Hay and Dr Sheppard had replaced him. Dr Sheppard's wife was also born in Ireland, and of a similar age to Dr Appleby's sister, but no direct connection between the two has been established.

BEAVAN (or BEVAN), Dr James.

Mr Beavan was a Surgeon-Captain in the Royal Radnorshire Militia and listed in 1780 as being of Hay and Bettws Clyro. A medical register for the year 1783 has him listed as Mr. Ja. Beavan of Hay. In 1785 Thomas Phillips of Chelsea took out an Apprentice Indenture for five years to Dr Beavan who was described as a surgeon and apothecary in Hay.

On the 24 July 1770 Dr Beavan married May Powell (baptised in 1744) the daughter of the Hay Excise Officer William Powell. A mortgage deed in Powys Record Office dated 2 March 1790 lists Dr Beavan as deceased but previously residing in Bridge Street (now Broad Street).

BOGLE, Dr Adam Linton, senior.

Dr Adam Linton Bogle senior was a surgeon living at Woodlands Glasbury between at least 1839 and 1859. He was the father of the well-known Hay G.P.

BOGLE, Dr Adam Linton, junior.

Dr Bogle worked at Pemberton House Surgery, but he and his wife Elizabeth lived at Henallt House 10/11 Oxford Road with their eight children.

- Two of their children died in infancy.
  Thomas Percy Templeton (28 July 1866-18 July 1867) and Augusta May (8–22 August 1869).
- Their son James H. who was born in 1852 and passed the preliminary examination of the Royal College of Physicians and Surgeons of Edinburgh on the 31 July 1866.[6] He was still in Scotland in 1871.
- John, who became a bank clerk was born in 1856. He married Ester Garthwaite in 1877.
- Sadly their son Adam Linton born 1858 was admitted to Bethlem Mental Hospital in 1882. He was discharged in 1892 but readmitted the following year and died in 1906.
- Kate M. was born in 1863.
- Adeline M. was born in 1868.
- Thomas L(inton) A(dam) was born in 1869.

There are a number of reports of Dr Bogle's busy medical career in Hay.

- He was called as a witness when a warrant was issued for the arrest of a Mr Reynolds on a charge of deserting his wife and leaving her destitute. At a hearing in October 1860 the defence council pointed out that she had left him. Mrs Reynolds retained possession of considerable property and 'instead of abusing her she had cruelly illtreated him'. Dr Bogle informed the Bench that 'he had seen Mr Reynold's body covered with bruises, said to have been inflicted by his wife'. Case dismissed.[7]
- Dr Bogle was involved in a court case against Charles Amos and another boy who threw stones at Victoria Meredith and her sister. On the 24 June 1866 George Haynes saw a stone they threw hit Victoria on the head. She began crying and lay down for a time. When she got up Charles hit her with another stone drawing blood. Dr Bogle found that Victoria had contusion and a wound penetrating through the scalp to the skull. Fortunately she recovered with no skin rash or infection. Charles was fined 12s 6d with 14s costs. Because his parents said they could not pay he was sentenced to 14 days in gaol.
- At the inquest of the butler Charles Ecclestone from Clyro Court in 1867 Dr Bogle described his findings at a post-mortem. The deceased had a burst blood vessel at the base of his brain, indicative of liver disease. Verdict natural causes.[8]

- As previously described Dr Bogle attended John Merrick the station porter who fell under the railway trucks at Hay railway station (see Accidents in Chapter 3).

Dr Bogle like many of the Victorian gentry volunteered in the local yeomanry. In his case he was appointed an Ensign in the 4th Breconshire Rifle Volunteer Corps on 30 July 1864.[9]

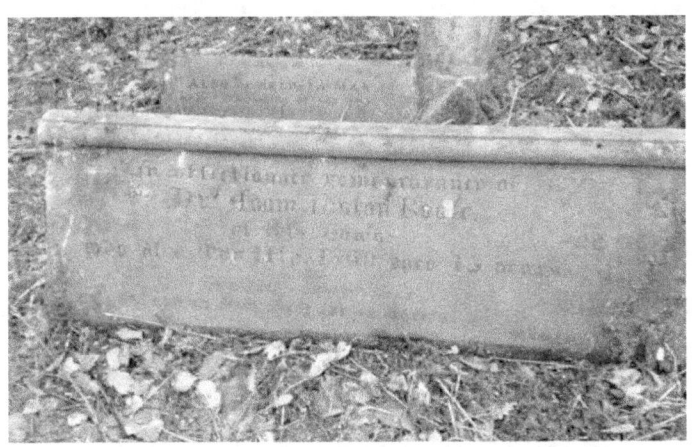

Dr Bogles grave marker in St Mary's churchyard.

After a busy fulfilling life Adam Linton Bogle died 11 May 1869 aged only 43 years. He left an estate valued at under £1,500.

BRIDGEWATER, Dr.

All that is known of Dr Bridgewater is that in 1853 he attended a patient who had been kicked in the stomach by his horse. The accident happened while he was out hunting with the Wyeside hounds so Dr Bridgewater may not have been a resident of Hay. Unfortunately the patient died 24hrs later.

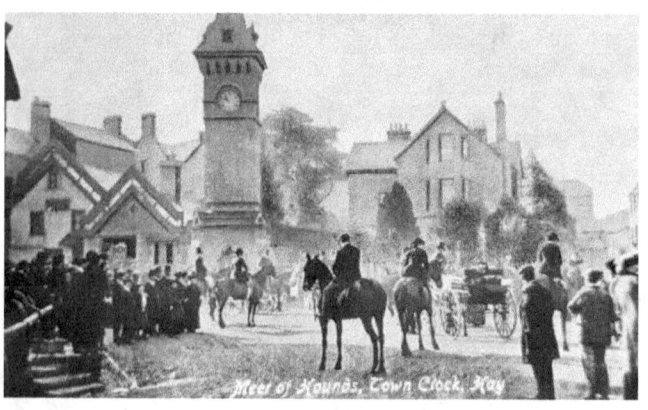

CAPLE, Dr Henry.

Dr Caple was born circa 1811 and listed as a surgeon of Castle Street in 1840.[10] In the 1841 census he was at 24 Broad Street so he may have moved to more prestigious premises, or Castle Street may have just been his surgery.

He was the first Medical Officer for Hay appointed by the Board of Guardians following the Poor Law Amendment Act of 1834. His tenure was short as he was not appointed before 1836 and had resigned by 1838.

Dr Caple and his wife Catherine had a son Arthur (born circa 1838). Sadly in 1842, despite the best efforts of Mr J.W.P. Lyde,[11] Catherine died suddenly after her supper from a fit of coughing which caused a blood vessel to burst.

CLOUSTON, Dr Charles Stewart. M.B., C.M., M.D.

Dr Clouston was born in 1847 on Sandwick in the Orkney Islands, the son of the distinguished surgeon and venerated father of the Church of Scotland the Rev. Dr Charles Clouston.

He was related to two old Norse Orkney families, the Traills of Holland and the Stewart's of Brugh, through his two grandmothers. His wife Emma (1848-1916) was the eldest daughter of William Traill M.D. of Orkney.

Dr Clouston studied medicine at Edinburgh University and was said to have a very scientific mind, always looking to improve his medical practice. He published a number of research papers.

After qualifying with honours in 1868 he moved to Hay and built an extensive practise. The Rev. Francis Kilvert noted in his dairy on 7 February 1872 that he was always being mistaken for Dr Clouston but recorded that he first met him on Tuesday 12 April 1870. Dr Clouston and Dr Trumper had just done a post-mortem examination on Matthew Lewis of Calva Farm Clyro. Lewis had died of a 'stoppage of the bowels' and their post-mortem showed he had a burst stomach ulcer.

Two days later Dr Clouston saw John Watkins of Castle Street and decided that 'from the wildness of his talk' he should be committed to the Talgarth asylum. Before issuing an order for his removal Dr Trumper, with the magistrate and the relieving officer, went to visit Watkins. On seeing them he appeared quite lucid and sane, so no order was issued.

Although Dr Clouston was appointed Medical Officer of Health in 1878 at £5 pa, and is recorded in Hay in Slaters Directory for 1880, he moved to Gunnersbury, London, that year. Here he successfully built a new practice. His work in rheumatism and the use of salicylates in his thesis led to a Doctorate in Medicine in 1881.[12]

In 1883 Dr Clouston suffered obscure hepatic and renal complications after a bout of pneumonia caused by catching scarlet fever from a patient.[13]

He went home to the Orkneys to recuperate in June of that year. Unhappily his health steadily declined, and he died aged 36 years on the 16 September. He left five young children, four daughters and one son, Charles, who died in Ficksburg South Africa 9 April 1902.

DICKSON, Dr T.G.

Other than his appointment as Medical Officer to Hay Local Board between 1897-99 nothing more is known of Dr Dickson.

EDWARDS, Mr.

He was employed as an assistant by Dr Reece in 1851, but again nothing more is known.

FEATHERSTONE, Dr George William Beaumont.

Dr Featherstone was an Australian born in Adelaide 14 July 1866. He qualified in 1891 and was working at Cadishead Manchester in the 1890's, marrying Mary Matilda Wills at Chapel-En-Le-Frith Derbyshire in 1897. Shortly afterwards he came to Hay and was appointed Medical Officer to the Local Board in 1899-1901.

In 1901 he was living in Pemberton House Bell Bank at the time Dr Lewis Heather was a visitor in the house. Dr Heather quickly took over the practice so on that basis Dr Featherstone does not appear to have practised in Hay for long, perhaps he was a long term locum.

By 1913 he was working in Aldershot, and died at Pentire, Newquay, Cornwall on 13 March 1934.[14]

GILES, Dr (Peter) Broome.

Dr Peter Broome Giles (born 1850), universally known as Dr Broome Giles, was the son of a doctor, also called Dr Peter Broome Giles. Dr Giles senior established a practice at Staunton upon Wye.

Dr Giles junior trained at University College London and qualified in 1871. It does not appear that he joined his father at Staunton after qualifying as at that time George Kenyon was employed as an assistant to his father.

Dr Giles junior quickly established his practice at Brobury. He was the designated Medical Officer of Health in Hay by 1876, at a salary of £1. 1s. 0d a day. His son, another Peter who also qualified as a doctor, was born at Brobury in 1884. By 1891 Dr Giles was employing Thomas Naylor as his assistant.

From the time he qualified Dr Giles took an active role in the Volunteer (military) movement and ambulance work. He became brigadier-surgeon lieutenant-colonel of the 1st Herefordshire Rifle Volunteers and Welsh Border Volunteer Infantry Brigade, and surgeon lieutenant-colonel in the Army Medical Reserve.

Whether it was through his medical or army careers, or a working holiday we do not know but he visited the continent in 1897. He published a letter in the British Medical Journal on the Walcher's position in obstetrics. In it he refers to eight skiagraphs, i.e. X-rays, he had taken in Germany. This was only one year after their discovery by William Roentgen.

Dr Giles was a keen follower of country sports. A keen shot and enthusiastic fisherman he was also Master of the Hereford Staghounds.

Around 1900, when he was 50 years old, Dr Giles left Brobury and settled in Buckinghamshire. He became a county councillor, county director of the London Branch of the Red Cross, and a colonel in the 1st London Division of the Territorial Force. During the First World War he was commandant of the military hospital at Alnwick and later Ashton-in-Makerfield.

In his army role he wrote books on the training of stretcher-bearers and papers on ambulance work and the training of medical units. He died in December 1928 aged 78 years.[15]

GRIFFITHS, Dr William A.

In 1881 William was a 17-year-old medical student but by 1891 Dr Griffiths was a surgeon and physician at Belle Vue House Broad Street.

HATHAWAY, Dr (Joseph) Nicholas.

Dr Hathaway had a practice in Wye Bridge Street (Broad Street) in 1830, probably at Tinto House 14 Broad Street where he was registered in the 1835 Pigot's Directory. By 1840 he was at 7 Castle Street according to Robson's Directory. In the 1841 census he was recorded as 37 years of age, so born about 1804.

By 1849 he had moved to Crich Derbyshire but before 1873 he had returned to live in Southbank House 21 Broad Street. Dr Hathaway was still in practice in 1881, again in Wye Bridge Street.

Dr Hathaway married Eliza Frances Howarth Davies, (baptised 3 May 1793 at Rotherhithe), on the 15 October 1829. They were married in Hay by the Rev. Morgan Walters. In 1838 the Rev. Walters died and Elizabeth inherited a share of his property including two swords, a night glass and telescope formerly the property of a relative, Admiral and Colonel Howarth.

On their marriage the couple borrowed £1000 from Eliza's aunt Mary Ann Norman wife of Captain Richard Norman. Sadly on 22 March 1839 Eliza died. Her will, dated 1838, discharged the loan from her aunt and also left £200 to each of their three children Norman Nicholas, Mary Ann Sarah and Frances Jane.

On the 11 September 1839 Dr Hathaway married again to Elizabeth Jones at St Mary le Bone.

On her death he went to live with his daughter Penelope in Weston Super Mare, where he died and was buried in 1883.

HEATHER, Dr Lewis Daniel. M.R.C.S. Eng., L.R.C.S. London.

Dr Heather was born in 1869. In 1901 he was a guest in Pemberton House but by 1911 he was the only doctor resident there. The 1910 Kelly's Directory records he was Medical Officer of Health to Hay Painscastle and Bredwardine Rural District Councils and Medical Officer and Public Vaccinator for Radnorshire.

On 18 July 1907 Dr Heather was called to an inquest at Clifford to confirm that Thomas Pritchard, labourer, had died of heatstroke while working in the fields.[16] Dr Heather died on 10 December 1912.

HIGGS, Dr.

Dr Higgs was described as a physician and surgeon in Hay when he took on an assistant Dr Charles Lewis in June 1879. A condition of his employment was that Dr Lewis would not practice medicine in Hay for 10 years after leaving Dr Higgs.

Just over one year later on 16 October 1880, and without the agreed one month's notice, Dr Higgs dismissed Lewis. Lewis promptly set up his own practice in the town. Dr Higgs applied to the High Court to prevent him doing this, and he was granted an injunction restraining the defendant until the hearing,[17] the results of which are unknown.

ACTION AGAINST A WELSH MEDICAL MAN.

In the High Court of Justice (Chancery Division) on Thursday, before Vice-chancellor Sir C. Hall, the case of Higgs v. Lewis came on for hearing. This was a motion on behalf of the plaintiff, Dr. Higgs, physician and surgeon, of Hay, Breconshire, to restrain the defendant Charles Lewis from practising as a medical man in the town or Hay or the neighbourhood. Mr Badcock said in June, 1879, Dr. Higgs engaged the defendant Charles Lewis to act as his assistant, and a written agreement was signed by both parties, which provided, amongst other things, that the agreement could be put an end to by a month's notice in writing, and that if the defendant left Dr. Higgs, he would not commence practice as a medical man in Hay or the neighbourhood for a period of ten years. The defendant acted as Dr. Higgs's assistant down to the 16th of October, 1880, when Dr. Higgs dismissed the defendant without the month's notice provided in the agreement. He read an affidavit of Dr. Higgs's, which, after stating the agreement and the defendant's dismissal, said that since the defendant had ceased to act as his assistant the defendant had commenced to practice in Hay and the neighbourhood.—There was no appearance on behalf of the defendant.

The Vice-Chancellor granted an injunction restraining the defendant from practising in Hay or the neighbourhood till the hearing of the action.

HINCKS FAMILY.

The Hincks family were a medical dynasty in Hay for over 50 years. The family consisted of Thomas senior, his wife Emily and their seven children, two of whom qualified as doctors.

HINCKS, Dr Thomas Samuel Hawkesford. M.D., C.M., J.P.

Dr Hincks senior was born in 1846 at Tettenhall Staffordshire. He came to Hay in 1875 shortly after his marriage in 1874 to Emily Fairbanks (born in 1850 in Walsall Staffordshire). In 1876 he was appointed the acting Assistant-Surgeon in the 4th Breconshire Rifle Volunteer Corps, replacing Dr Joseph Evans Smith.[18]

The first record of them living at Cartrefle, now called Tinto House, no.13 Broad Street was in 1881. Dr Hincks surgery was next door at no.14. His higher degree of Doctor of Medicine from the University of Edinburgh was published in the British Medical Journal in 1885.[19]

Dr Hincks was a traditional old fashioned country doctor who had a reputation as a firm but kind clinician. He was a stalwart member of the Hay community for 50 years.

In the days before the motor car he found it necessary to keep a number of horses. These were essential to enable him to ride extensively over the hills to see his patients.

Dr Hincks was appointed Medical Officer and Public Vaccinator to Hay Union, and Medical Officer to the Workhouse after Dr Smith resigned.[20] In 1875 he was elected an Urban District Councillor[21] and by 1904 was a Brecon County Councillor.

In 1914 he became one of the Justices under the Lunacy Act 1890 i.e able to make Reception Orders (admit a patient to a mental asylum). At the beginning of the First World War, as the most senior local doctor, he gave at least two lectures to the Hay Voluntary Aid Detachment.

Dr Hincks was also one of the six canvassers for volunteers for the forces. On the 25 November 1915 he reported that the town canvassers had forwarded their recruitment blue cards for men in the town aged between 18 and 41 years.

In his spare time he was a keen tennis player and an enthusiastic chrysanthemum grower.

His wife Emily had her share of the typical Victorian doctors wife 'good works'. In addition to her church work she supported the Girls Friendly Society Zenana Missions, and the Hay and Cusop Nursing Association. She predeceased her husband on 5 January 1925 shortly after their golden wedding anniversary. Dr Hincks died on the 11 June 1930 aged 85yrs.

Two of their sons followed their father into the medical profession.

HINCKS, Dr Thomas Ernest. M.D., Ch. B.

Their eldest son, known as Tom, was born in April 1876. He qualified in medicine at Edinburgh and worked briefly in Birmingham before joining his father in Hay, and where he practiced as a G.P. for 34 years.

A man of great charm, Dr Tom was widely respected in the town and popular. When he returned by train from his honeymoon in 1907 'bringing his lovely young bride back to Hay' a pony and trap were waiting for them. A group of 'young blades' unhitched the horses and got between the shafts, pulling the couple up Ship Pitch and Castle Street, then down Oxford Road to their new home at no.9.

Dr Tom was often seen on horseback riding out to visit patients on hill farms in all weathers, sometimes with his wife Laura (born in Bexhill on Sea) accompanying him in a trap.

He succeeded his father in many appointments. At the 1910 council meeting he was appointed certifying surgeon under the Factory and Workshop Acts[22] and the Medical Officer for the Bredwardine and Painscastle Rural District Council. At the same meeting he was also reappointed as Medical Officer for Hay at £5 p.a. with fees of £1.17s.6d.

Dr Tom gave evidence to the Hay Urban District Council on 8 June 1916 regarding the call up of garage mechanic Ernest Knight. Ernest was employed by Mr Webb of Lion Street who said his garage would be useless to his clients without a mechanic. Dr Tom and Dr Shepherd testified it was essential that a motor car and garage should be kept going for them to do their work. Dr Tom also stated that if, or more likely when, he was called up to the R.A.M.C. it would be essential that a locum doctor had the support of a driver who knew the district.

Twenty years earlier on the 5 August 1896 Dr Tom had joined the 1st (Brecknockshire) Volunteer

Battalion South Wales Borderers as a Second Lieutenant. After the army reorganisation on the 1 April 1908, he was appointed as a captain in a supernumerary capacity in the Brecknockshire Battalion South Wales Borderers. Sure enough, as the First World War raged, he was called up. On the 30 November 1916 he was commissioned into the R.A.M.C. with the rank of captain.

After spending Christmas at home he left for war shortly afterwards. It was reported in May 1917 that he had arrived in Mesopotamia and handed the duties of medical officer of the surgical ward at the General Hospital at Amara. In January 1918 he returned home after just under a year at Amara and a short time in India and Egypt.

On the 19 December 1922 the War Office recorded that Temporary Captain Thomas Ernest Hincks M.B. Royal Army Medical Corps had been awarded the Medaille des Epidemics, en Bronze.[23] This medal was awarded for services supporting the French Health Service in 1918 containing contagious disease.

As would be expected Dr Tom had many memorable events during his years of practice. One might have been when he was called to attend the Rev. G. Dermer Pagden of Cusop. On entering his pulpit to deliver his Sunday sermon in December 1900, Rev. Pagden said 'Dearly Beloved' then collapsed and died.[24]

Grwyne Fawr Dam.

In 1913 Dr Tom was appointed as the medical officer and panel doctor, at £50 per annum, to the navies living at Blaen-y-Cwm. This was a camp in the

Black Mountains for the workers who were building the new Grwyne Fawr Dam and reservoir. Dr Tom reported 'the present nursing arrangements are most satisfactory', but due to the isolation of the site he suggested a 'Blaen-y-cwm and District General Hospital' be set up. He then went off to war.

Work on the dam largely shut down during the hostilities but in 1919 it recommenced. A small village of approximately 400 people grew up down the valley from the dam. It had a school, shop, and police station. Dr Tom was reappointed medical officer in June 1919.

Before the war he had visited on horseback, riding the ten miles over the hills from Hay twice a week. After the war he went by car each Tuesday to Pont Esgob, and then by the 3ft gauge steam railway to the camp.

Dr Tom employed a 'French' war widow as a chauffeuse according to Miss Lilwall of Hay. The chauffeuse was English so possibly her husband was a French soldier. Dr Tom was not noted for his punctuality and the company complained it had to pay considerable overtime to train drivers due to this.

All medical services were his responsible and he appointed nurses to run the hospital - Sister Thorne, followed by Sister McKenzie, Nurse Mytton, Sister Whitney and Nurse Williams. Sister Kinsey from Hay also attended on occasions. There was an isolation hospital and a train carriage was fitted out as an ambulance but it is not known if either were used.

That medical facilities were needed was demonstrated by Dr Tom when he informed the company in 1925 that his work had doubled, and he had to spend £100 on drugs when the allowance was only £30.

The Armstrong Poisoning

In many ways Dr Tom's legacy was the national prominence, and damaged reputation, he acquired at the trial of the Hay solicitor Herbert Rowse Armstrong.

Following chemist Fred Davies' suspicions of arsenic poisoning it was Dr Tom who contacted the Home Office. This ultimately led to the conviction of Armstrong for the murder of his wife Katherine.[25]

Dr Tom Ernest Hincks 'died on the 8 November 1932 aged 57 years thirty four years medical practitioner in this town' following a heart attack while riding on Penshigley Hill, Cusop. Ironically this was within sight of Herbert Armstrong's house.

Dr Tom had two sons who died during the Second World war.

- Lieutenant Thomas Stuart Hincks 238387 was born on 20 June 1907. He was appointed to the General Army List Ceylon Pioneer Battalion attached to the Ceylon Auxiliary Pioneer Battalion on the 3 April 1942.[26] He was killed on the 2 November 1943 and is commemorated on the Trincomalee War Cemetery Sri Lanka.
- His brother 2nd Lieutenant John Hawkesford Hincks 79908 was born 22 October 1910 and attended Bromsgrove School 1924-28. A member of the 5th Cinque Ports Battalion of the Royal Sussex regiment he was killed 27-29 May 1940

during the defence of Dunkirk. He is buried in the Caestre Communal Cemetery France.

HINCKS, Dr (Arthur) Cecil M.B., M.C., Ch.B.

Cecil was born in 1882 and like his brothers went to Christ Church College Brecon. He qualified as a doctor in Birmingham and in 1908 he set up practice in Wells, Somerset.

At the beginning of the First World War Dr Cecil joined the 26th Field Ambulance which left for France as part of 8th Division British Expeditionary Force. His detailed letters described the working conditions, such as on the 13th and 19th of December to clear the hospital in readiness for new batches of casualties. Despite this they managed to put on a concert on Boxing Day. Dr Cecil was mentioned in despatches by Sir John French in 1914, and awarded the Military Cross the following year.[27]

HAY DOCTOR'S DISTINCTION. LIEUTENANT HINCKS.

The announcement in the 'London Gazette' of April 25th that His Majesty the King has been graciously pleased to confer the Military Cross on Lieut. A.C. Hincks, amongst other officers, in recognition of his gallantry and devotion to duty whilst serving with the Expeditionary Force, will give the greatest satisfaction to all Breconions and particularly to the people of Hay and the surrounding district. Lieut. A.C. Hincks is the son of Dr T.S.H. Hincks, of Hay, and brother to the better known Dr Tom Hincks. He was educated at Christ College, Brecon, where the news of his distinction has been received with feelings of great pride. Entering the medical profession he became house surgeon and house physician at the Birmingham General Hospital, and in 1908 began practising at Wells, later entering into partnership with Drs Allen and Smith. At the outbreak of the war he offered his services and was attached to the 4th Somersets, but before they left for India he was transferred to the 4th Wilts, and later to an ambulance corps at Torquay. He was once again transferred, this time to the 26th Field Ambulance R.A.M.C., Territorial Force (2nd Wessex), stationed in Hampshire. On Nov. 5th he left for France, where he has since been carrying out medical duties. Towards the end of February, says the 'Somerset and West of England Advertiser,' he obtained five days' leave and returned to WSIIP, but he was very reticent as to the fighting he had witnessed. It was ascertained, however, that even up to that time he had had many exciting experiences and narrow escapes. The King's mark of recognition of the gallant Lieutenant's bravery is recorded in the 'London Gazette' under the heading of 'The Military Cross' and in the following terms 'Lieut. A.C. Hincks, 26th Field Ambulance, R.A.M.C., Territorial Force (2nd Wessex). - For conspicuous gallantry and devotion to duty at Neuve Chapelle from March 11th to 14th, 1915, in collecting the wounded whilst under heavy fire. On the night of March 13-14, whilst he was attending to a wounded man, a shell struck the ambulance waggon, killing the man and rendering Lieut. Hincks unconscious. On recovering he at once proceeded to collect the wounded under fire, and continued doing so throughout the morning.'

Brecon County Times (6 May 1915).

Following the Battle of Neuve-Chapelle he was again mentioned in despatches as well as obtaining a D.S.O. Lt Cecil wrote letters home describing his experiences in France and exerts have been published by the Hay History Group.[28] In 1917 he was promoted captain.

After the war Dr Cecil resumed his practice and became the Medical Officer of Health in Wells and senior physician in the cottage hospital. He served in many roles locally and nationally for the British Medical Association, and was a member of the Local Medical War Committee. During the 2nd World War he was a major in the Home Guard and an Air Raid Precautions lecturer and instructor.

Dr Cecil married Mrs Ethel Florence McGillycuddy on the 28 January 1921. She was the widow of Major Richard Hugh McGillycuddy R.A.M.C. who died 21st October 1918 and is buried in Netley Military Cemetery, Southampton.[29]

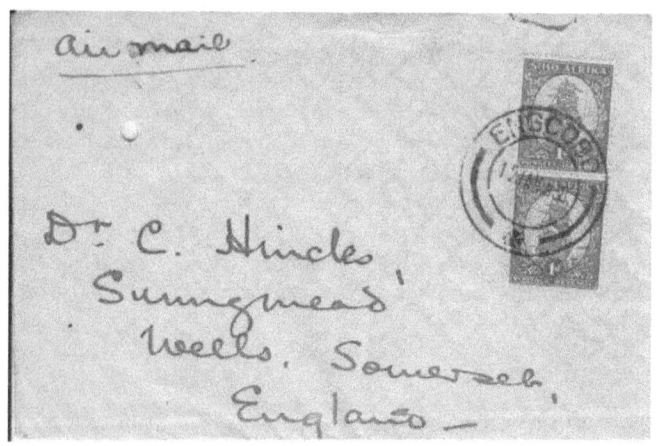

Ethel and Cecil lived at Sunnymead, St Thomas Street, Wells and had two sons Michael and Peter. Dr Cecil died 26 August 1949 at Wells Cottage Hospital. His obituary notes the affection the city held for their long serving medic.[30]

The other Hincks children did not follow the family medical tradition.

- Edwyn Hawksford Hereford Hincks was born 10 June 1877 and died 18 December 1913.

- William Harvey Hincks, born 1878, joined the Pembrokeshire Imperial Yeomanry for active service in the 2nd Boer War in February 1900. He was presented with a belt, purse and money by his friends in Hay. The National Provincial Bank in Brecon gave him a service revolver and the manager Mr Bradley presented a service knife. South Africa must have agreed with William as 20 years later he was still there in the Cape Mounted Rifles. He married Pearl Edith Sofia Cook and they settled in Umtata, the capital of Cape Colony. They had two children – Cecil Hawkesford and Alan Philip. William died at Umtata 26 January 1921, during the great drought, 'as a result of the hardships of the war'.[31]
- Harold Austin Hincks was born in 1881 and like his brother served in the Boer War in the 30 (Pembrokeshire) Company 9th Battalion Imperial Yeomanry. After a one-year short service attestation he returned in February 1901, and then went to Canada in 1903. He returned and married Nora Johnson at King's Heath Birmingham in 1912. They emigrated to Canada going via Liverpool to New York. In 1916 their only child Eileen was born in Victoria, British Columbia.
- (Emily) Dorothy Mary Hincks was born in 1886 and assisted her father with the dispensing of medicines. She retained a medical connection by marrying Dr (Francis) Richard Todd of North Petherton, Somerset on the 19 February 1917. They moved to Heathfield House in Creech St

Michael Somerset. Dr Todd died in 1931 but Dorothy went on to train as a nurse and lived until 1 June 1954.

- Bertram Hincks was born 1 May 1890 and went to Christ Church College like his brothers. He also went to Canada, apparently to visit his brother Harold A.,[32] and shortly afterwards he was reported to have emigrated to British Columbia. Not long afterwards he was apparently poultry farming in California.[33] Immediately on the outbreak of war he volunteered and returned to fight in France as a private in the 16th Battalion British Columbian Highland Regiment with the Canadian Expeditionary Force.

    They landed at Plymouth and were billeted on Salisbury Plain before embarked for France. On the 6 May 1915 Bertram took part in the Colonials 'brilliant charge' at the second Battle of Ypres and the subsequent fighting at Festubert. By 23 September 1915 Lance-Corporal Hincks was at home for a short leave.

    After returning to the front in France he came back in the spring of 1916 to take up a commission. Attached to the Cambridge Officer Training Corps for training he was gazetted in June as a 2nd Lt Kings Royal Rifle Corps. By October 1916 he was qualified as a sniping officer. While doing his rounds at Morval on the 17 December 1916 2nd Lt Hincks of the 5th Battalion attached to the 10th Battalion K.R.R.C. was shot in the head and killed.

He was 26 years old.[34] His grave is in Delville Wood Cemetery Longueval, Somme, France.

Members of the Hincks family are recorded on a memorial in St Mary's graveyard Hay. Dr Thomas (Snr) Hincks, his wife Emily, Edwyn, William Harvey who died in South Africa, Bertram who died in the First World War, and John and Thomas the sons of Dr Tom Hincks who were killed in the Second World War.

JARVIS, Dr James.
Dr James Jarvis is mentioned in the Hay churchwardens rate book of 1825 but no other details known.

JONES, Dr John.
The Hay parish records of 14 February 1730 show that a John Jones surgeon was implored 'to use his best endeavour to recover Eliz. James to her former senses being at present very ill'.

Fifty years later in 1780 a Dr John Jones was listed as a surgeon-apothecary. He is also listed in the medical register for the year 1783 as working in Hay, and was still alive in 1792. Dr Jones was paid £5 11s 0d on 6 March 1781 to attend David James a tinkers son who had been shot by William Powell.

An undated gravestone in St Mary's Churchyard may be his as it reads '...of this town, Surgeon, 76 years'. His tombstone features skull and crossbones and was 'made by John Millward'.

LEWIS, Dr Charles.

Dr Charles Lewis was employed as an assistant in the practice of Dr Higgs in 1879. After his dismissal without the contractual one month's notice he set up in practice in Hay against the original terms of his employment contract. Dr Higgs took him to court to stop him. (see Dr Higgs above).

LEWIS, Dr James.

Dr James Lewis was a surgeon and apothecary in Hay. Born in 1760 he is mentioned as a beneficiary in the Lewis Family Papers dated August 1798 at the Powys Record Office.

He died on the 12 August 1827[35] and is buried in plot 102 St Mary's Church, Cusop.

LYDE, Dr James Watkins Price.

From the dates it seems there were three doctors of different generations with this distinctive name. In all likelihood fathers and sons.

- The first Dr James Watkins Price Lyde, was listed as a surgeon-apothecary in 1780, and in a medical register for 1783. In 1791 Williams Symonds started an apprenticeship with him.[36] Dr Lyde married Elizabeth Watkins on 11 June 1782.

  A Dr Lyde is named in the manorial court of 1776 as an offender when the court was prosecuting individuals for having dunghills outside their houses in the street. This must have been him. Possibly the dunghill was outside his surgery which could have been at 3 or 4 Church Street, where his son lived and had his surgery later. Dr Lyde senior died in 1861 aged 99 years.

In 1801 this Dr Lyde inherited the use of Lower House, Cusop, for a period of 14 years, together with numerous other properties, from his father-in-law Thomas Watkins. These included Llangwatham House and Mill with 2 wheels, the Pant, Pontybaker, flannel mill and Margaret's Garden, and numerous fields around Hay shown on the 1846 Tythe Survey.

Prior to this he must have had the use of these properties as he advertised them for rent in January 1791. A reward was also offered for the return of his bay gelding, lost or stolen, in September 1799. In September 1812 he was again advertising to let a woollen manufactory and tucking mill half a mile from Hay, near his mill in Cusop Dingle. In 1806 a piece of land known as Lydes Meadow was auctioned and this cannot have been unconnected to him.

In 1801 the will of Thomas Watkins left land to both his son in law J.W.P. Lyde (senior), and also to his grandson (see below) who was also called James Watkins Price Lyde. This land was in the area of Peterchurch, Dorstone and Cusop.

- A second James Watkins Price Lyde was born in 1784 and is listed as a surgeon in London in 1820. In 1830 a surgeon of this name was at The George in Hay but Piggotts Directories for 1835 and 1840 place his surgery at no.3 Church Street with him living next door at no.4. Later census returns record him as a 57-year-old surgeon in 1841, a 65 year old surgeon in 1851 and a 77 year old G.P. Surgeon M.R.C.S. in 1861. Dr Lyde was a signatory to the Herefordshire Memorandum in 1845 (see Dr Thomas).

In 1851 the second J.W.P. Lyde had a large pair of scissors stolen from him, for which Henry Hanright was sentenced to three months in Brecon gaol.[37]

Dr Lyde was also one of only twelve householders to pay a tithe rent on his land in Hay.[38] In 1853, along with Dr Bridgewater and Mr Reece, he attended William Lewis who later died after he was kicked in the stomach by his horse while out hunting with the Wyeside hounds. This Dr Lyde died on 2 April 1869 in St Pancras, Camden, London aged 85years.

- Eight months after the above J.W.P. Lyde died an indenture dated 2 December 1869 states a J.W.P. Lyde held surgery at no.3 Church Street and lived next door at no.4 Church Street. This would be his son. The Piggotts Directory for 1881 records this third J. Lyde, and grandson of the surgeon-apothecary of 1780, practicing in Castle Street.

One of the second two J.W.P. Lyde's would have been the one recorded at Talgarth in 1832 and Peterchurch in 1852 and 1857.

On 16 August 1804 a Dr James Lyde attended the inquest of an illegitimate female child, the victim of infanticide by Mary Morris. Mary was a servant to James Watkin. He may have been the saddler in Castle Street, and not related or to be confused with Thomas Watkins Dr Lydes father-in-law.

Mary killed her new-born with a pair of scissors and hid the body in a potato field. It was quickly discovered. Mary was found not guilty of murder but guilty of 'concealment of birth' for which she was given 2 years hard labour at Brecon Assizes. This was in stark contrast to the tragic case of Mary Morgan of Llowes who was hanged at Presteigne for a similar offence a few months later.[39]

The doctor involved was the elder Dr Lyde who would have been 42 years old rather than his son who was only 18 years at the time.

The Hereford Times of 19 January 1848 records a Mr Lyde was called to attend Thomas Mabe aged 16 years following an assault by a fellow servant at the local butcher's where they worked. He had received a number of blows to his head. Mr Lyde advised his mother to apply a dozen leeches to the head wound.

The next day he examined Thomas and found only light bruising but otherwise he was well. Thomas gradually became ill over the next 3 days, and a week after the assault he died. Mr Lyde did a post-mortem which found a skull fracture, a broken blood vessel and coagulated blood, i.e. what we would now call a subdural haematoma.

This is unlikely to have been Dr Lyde senior as in 1848 he would have been 88 years old, but could have been his son of 64 years, or his grandson of 45 years.

MOLOHAN, Dr Michael Henry.

Dr Molohan was a member of a large family from Tromora House in Ireland.

In 1881 he was a 26-year-old assistant physicians surgeon at 14 Broad Street. This became the surgery of Dr Thomas S.H. Hincks who moved to Hay at this time. Possibly Dr Molohan covered Dr Hathaway leaving and Dr Hincks arriving.

By 1885 Dr Molohan had established his own practice at Towcester.[40] He died on the 1 April 1897 at the age of 43 years, and is commemorated on a family memorial at Kilmurry-Ibrickane, Mullage, County Clare, Ireland.

OWENS, Dr David Price.

Dr Owens was born in 1790 and recorded as a surgeon at Brook House, Water Street (now Heol y Dwr) in 1840.

The newspapers reported Dr Owens:

'performed an excellent and surprising cure on the child of Mr Shaw Superintendent of Police'. The child had a substance formed under the tongue, and which prevented it from speaking so as to be understood, although at the time the case was submitted to Mr Owens, it was more than three years old. Mr O. undertook to perform a cure, and after attending to it for about three months the child was enabled to speak plainly, the cure being effected without the assistance of any instrument'.[41]

Sadly Dr Owens died before his daughters marriage in 1860.

PAUL, Dr.
Dr Paul was a G.P. in Hay during the second World War.

POWELL, Dr Hubert (Hugh) Wyebrands L.R.C.P. Edin. M.R.C.S. Eng.
Dr Powell was a physician and surgeon, and Medical Officer and Public Vaccinator for Radnorshire District Hay Union.[42] Originally he was in partnership with Dr Tom Hincks but he moved to Pemberton House in 1919 and had his surgery there until 1955.

His grave marker records he was for 35 years a 'Beloved Physician in this Place 22.9.1882–27.2.1955'.

PRICE, Dr Daniel.
A tombstone in St Mary's Churchyard Hay records 'Here lieth the body of Daniel Price of this town, surgeon, who departed this life 2 (May) 1767 aged 34 years'.

PRICE, Dr David Owen.
Piggotts Directory 1881 lists Dr David Price as a surgeon in Red Lion Street, (one end of the present Lion Street). No other record can be found of him in Hay for that year so this may have been his surgery and he could have lived outside the town.

PRICE, Dr Henry.

In December 1845 a Dr Henry Price, surgeon of Hay, was called to examine the body of William Price a 16-year-old farm worker found collapsed below the wheel of a threshing machine. The Hereford Journal reported that Dr Price found that he was 'quite dead. On examination he saw a small contusion on each side of his head, with a fracture of the skull'.[43]

No records can be found to confirm Dr Price lived in the Hay area.

PRICE, Dr Rees.

Dr Rees Price, described as a surgeon of Hay, was a witness to the assignment of a number of leases in October 1772. A piece of land he rented in Hay for £3 5s. 0d. was auctioned off in December 1798.[44] He may also have been the owner of a large number of oak trees for sale by auction at Brecon in 1807.

PROCTOR, Dr E.

Piggott's Medical Register of 1830 lists a Dr E. Proctor of Wye Bridge Street, (now Broad Street) and the 1830 Piggott's Directory lists Proctor and Son surgeons. By 1835 the directory only records a Henry Proctor so Dr E. Proctor must have retired or died.

PROCTOR, Dr Henry.

Dr Henry Proctor was born around 1795 and lived at 8 Broad Street from at least 1833. He was appointed surgeon to the Rose and Crown Amicable Society between at least 1843 and 1850.[45]

- Hay was not short of public houses, and these were a constant source of work for the doctors. In 1833 Dr Proctor was called to see Thomas Williams at the Blue Boar Inn. Williams had provoked and taunted Samuel Vaughan to a fight, as a consequence of which Williams was beaten and fell to the ground. He was in an exhausted state when Dr Proctor examined him and died shortly afterwards. The death certificate stated death was due to the fall. Vaughan was indited, but despite the judge directing the jury to find a verdict of manslaughter, they found him not guilty.[46]
- Thomas Evans was a boy with a team of timber hauliers who fell and was run over by their wagon. The hauliers were staying in the Nelson public house by the railway station overnight and did not see the accident. They ignored Thomas' absence, as well as an account of him being seen in a ditch.

    The next morning his father borrowed a horse and cart from the landlord and went to look for his son. He found him with injuries including fractures to his right foot and left elbow, compound fractures to his arm, and a deep laceration to his thigh. Thomas was conveyed to the workhouse infirmary where Dr Proctor did what he could but Thomas died 3 days later.[47]
- On the 1 March 1866 Dr Proctor resigned as Medical Officer to the Hay Union after serving in that capacity for 30 years. A typical example of the type of duties he would be involved in at the workhouse occurred in 1862. Mr Tasker, overseer

to the parish of Hay, applied for John Jones and his wife Alice to be removed from Hay to his place of birth, Shelsley Beaucham in Worcestershire. This was due to his infirmity and consequent admittance to the Hay Workhouse. Edward Powell the relieving officer for the workhouse confirmed that supporting him was a drain on parish funds. In court Dr Proctor, as surgeon to the workhouse, attested to the permanent nature of Jones illness. As a consequence Jones was ordered to return to Shelsley where they would be responsible for his welfare.[48]

- Dr Proctor officially retired from practice 25 March 1866. His work was then divided between Dr Bogle and Dr Smith.[49] Despite this on the 2 August 1867 he was called to attend to Charles Price, a mason who fell down the stairs of one of the Gwynne Almshouses in Chain Alley, Wyeford Road at about 1.00p.m. Price was in a state of drunkenness and sustained a wound to the back of the head. He died six hours later.

Dr Proctor married Elizabeth, possibly also known as Annie, who was born in 1801 in Hay. They had two sons and two daughters.

- Henry Richard, born 1818, was described as a druggist in 1851 and still living at home. He emigrated to Australia where he was elected mayor of Smythesdale in Victoria in 1878.[50]
- Richard who became a chemist in Penarth.[51]

- Eliza Ann and Margaret Jane married brothers James and Edward Hodges on the 18 April 1857.[52]

Dr Proctor's grave marker records '....for nearly half a century Surgeon of this place who died 24th September 1869 in his 76th year'.[53]

PUGH, Dr Thomas.
The only reference to Dr Pugh is in Piggott's Commercial Directory 1881 when he was listed as working in Black Lion Street.

REECE, Dr Ebenezer.
Dr Reece was in Oxford Road in 1839, (Slaters Directory), Prospect Terrace in 1840 and 1844, (Piggott's Directory), and Bronith Cottage in 1854, (Slaters Directory). Dr Reece employed at least one assistant. In 1851 he was a Mr Edwards who attended an accident when Mr Kentish the Superintendent of Hay Police was seriously injured after his horse threw him.[54]

By 1858 Dr Reece had moved to Oxford Road, (Slaters Directory), but by 1860 he was noted as formerly of Hay.[55] For some reason all his household effects had been auctioned off on the 25 May 1848.[56]

- Dr Reece was a member of the Independent Order of Oddfellows and in 1842 he was 'paid a very handsome tribute .... For his skilful and humane treatment of a poor girl .... in a dangerous and difficult operation'.[57]

- Six years later the inquest into the death of John Morgan from Moiety near Llowes gave great credit to Dr Reece for unravelling a mystery. John was found in a ditch. Dr Reece unravelled the story of how a gun exploded and killed him, and how his friend, so frightened by the accident, carried the body and hid it in a ditch.[58]
- In 1853 he attended, with Drs Bogle and Bridgewater, to William Lewis who had been kicked in the stomach by his horse while out hunting with the Wyeside hounds.[59]

SHEPHERD, Dr Robert John. L.C.R.P.

Dr Shepherd was born in Ireland in 1853 and graduated as a Licentiate of the King's and Queen's College of Physicians (Ireland).

There is no record of when he arrived in Hay. He was registered at Pembertons in 1891 and in the 1895 Kelly's directory. His predecessor at Pembertons Dr Appleby also came from Ireland, so there may have been a connection.

Dr Shepherd soon established himself. He became the Physician and Medical Officer of Health to the Local Board and Rural Sanitary Authority for the Urban and Rural District Councils, Medical Officer and Public Vaccinator Radnorshire District, as well as Medical Officer to Hay Union. All this despite Dr Thomas Hincks arriving in Hay five or six years before him. Dr Sheppard left Hay in 1919.

- Dr Shepherd was admonished by the Local Board on a number of occasions due to his poor attendance at committee meetings of the Hay Union, which he seems never to have attended.
- He attended Dr Williams of Talgarth at the time of his death in July 1914.
- On the 8 June 1916 he gave evidence to the Hay Urban District Council regarding the call up of garage mechanic Ernest Knight. Mr Webb of Lion Street said his garage would be useless to his clients without his mechanic Ernest. Dr Shepherd together with Dr Tom Hincks testified it was essential that a motor car and the garage should be kept going to enable them to do their rounds.

SMITH, Dr.

A Dr Smith is mentioned in a court leet of 1727. No other details known.

SMITH, Dr Joseph Evans.

Dr Smith was born around 1821, qualified in surgery in 1855[60] and medicine in 1856.[61]

In July 1866 he was appointed surgeon to the Hay branch of the Ancient Order of Foresters in Oxford Road. In 1871 his address was Henault House 11 Oxford Road, the house of Dr Bogle ten years earlier. In 1872 he was the Medical Officer to the Hay Union.

- At an inquest June 1866 Dr Smith certified that a tradesman John Blanden Newman a grocer in

Castle Street who fell down dead, died of 'paralysis of the nerves of the heart' i.e. a heart attack.[62]

- Dr Smith also attended an inquest to certify the death of Philip Pembridge, a tailor in Hay. He died after falling down his cellar steps in a state of intoxication in August 1869.

TAYLOR, Dr Henry.

There are a number of references to a surgeon of this name in Hay. These suggest two people.

- Dr Henry Taylor who died in 1826.

An advert in the Hereford Journal August 1819 names a Dr Henry Taylor as the representative of the executrix of the will of George Games of Clyro.

In December 1826 Dr Taylor's wife placed another advertisement. This time she was the executrix of her husband's will and asked for payment of any of his outstanding accounts.

A Dr Henry Taylor is also referred to on a gravestone in St Mary's graveyard Hay recording his wife Sarah's death on 1 January 1828 aged 45 years.

- Dr Henry Bayley Taylor surgeon, formerly of Hay, who died in 1855 in Cheltenham.

His birth is given as 1786[63] but nothing else is known about him. His widow died 7 March 1866 aged 57 years making her birth about 1809.

While no details have been found to corroborate the two Dr Taylors were father and son from the dates and similar names it is just possible that they were.

TAYLOR, Dr John Charles.

A tombstone in St Marys graveyard to Dr John Charles Taylor states he was for 'many years surgeon and apothecary in this town in which capacity, as well as in private life, he was well esteemed by all that knew him'.

The River Wye can be dangerous even in summer. Unfortunately Dr Taylor was drowned fording the river five miles upstream from Hay between Boughrood and Ripton on the 5 June 1825. He was 45 years old.[64]

THOMAS, Mr Joseph.

Piggott's directories list Mr Joseph Thomas as a surgeon living in Church Street in 1840 and 1844.

In April 1845 he, with Dr F. Trumper and Dr J.W.P. Lyde, was a signatory to the Herefordshire Memorandum. This was a petition by G.P.'s from Radnorshire, Breconshire and Herefordshire protesting to the terms of the recent Charter of Incorporation of the Royal College of Surgeons. They wished to be allowed to become Fellows based on length of registration rather than the whim of the committee of the College. This was part of a national protest by G.P.'s which led to changes incorporating their views.[65]

TRUMPER, Dr Francis Robert.

Dr Francis Trumper was a G.P. and surgeon, magistrate and landowner. His father Francis had the middle name Walwyn. Sir Thomas Walwyn was a Norman knight who is associated with a castle in Hay around 1120, and whose descendants stayed in the town for centuries. Use of this unusual name suggests that the Trumpers may have been an old Hay family.

Dr Trumper was born in 1819, and by 1851 was living at 66 Church Street. He was first registered as a member of the Royal College of Surgeons of England on 29 April 1842, and he was in their first national medical register issued in 1845.

Despite this we know he was practicing before then. In 1838 he gave evidence at the inquest into the sudden death of James Makin. Makin had awoken in the night, taken a drink of tea, started violent retching and then collapsed. As a result of Dr Trumper's medical evidence a verdict of 'Died by the visitation of God' was recorded.[66]

Dr Trumper was also a signatory to the Herefordshire Memorandum in 1845 (see Dr Thomas). By 1861 he was listed not only as a member of the Royal College of Surgeons but also a Licentiate of Apothecaries Hall, i.e. a registered apothecary.

In 1871 his address was Brook House, 6 Brook Street, where he lived his remaining years. He had married Emma Bevan, nee Higgins in 1854, and Brook House may have been her family home. Sadly she died in 1865 aged only 49 years. Dr Trumper endowed the marble pulpit in St Mary's Church Hay in memory of his wife and his mother-in-law Fortune Higgs.

Dr Francis Trumper died 14 November 1913 and is buried in Dorstone cemetery. His will dated 20 June 1913 is in the deeds of 4 Church Street Hay. The street has been renumbered so the present no.4 may have been the no.66 where he was living in 1851.

TRUMPER, Dr Hubert Bagster.

Dr Hubert Bagster Trumper was the son of the distinguished Birmingham G.P. Dr Oscar Bagster Trumper. Dr Oscar bought the land on which the ruins of Clifford Castle sit and erected his retirement home in its grounds.

Dr Hubert was born in 1902 at Market Raisin, Lincolnshire. When he qualified in 1926 he joined his father as a G.P. in Birmingham. Skin pigmentation in some of his patients led him to investigate skin disease caused by industrial process'. This interest led him to become the medical officer to the Association of British Chromium Depositors in 1931, and he published an article in the B.M.J. on the dangers of this work the same year.[67]

At the outbreak of World War Two Dr Trumper evacuated his family from Birmingham to the safety of the house his father had built at Clifford.

In 1928 he had joined the Territorial Army, and on the outbreak of war in 1939 he went with the British Expeditionary Force to France. As a lieutenant colonel in the Royal Army Medical Corps (145th Field Ambulance) he spent the winter in France, partly on the Maginot Line. The Dunkirk evacuation was a very traumatic time for him but he managed to arrive home safely with the troops.

(For an excellent account of the confusing conditions they experienced see Norman Smith's memoirs.[68])

For the rest of the war Dr Trumper worked for Imperial Chemical Industries (I.C.I.). They requested his help to develop treatment for the skin of persons who had been exposed to radiation. This was all part of Project Manhattan, the development of the atomic bomb.

After the war he was personnel manager at I.C.I. from 1946 to 1949 but left due to a difference of opinion with Dr Amit who also worked at the plant. Dr Trumper was concerned that certain process' exposed workers to risk of cancer, in conflict with the views of Dr Amit. He was unsuccessful in suing I.C.I. for unfair dismissal.[69]

On leaving I.C.I. Dr Trumper became a G.P. in Hay. He joined Dr Walter (William) Wilson at the surgery at Tinto House 13 Broad Street in 1949. In 1959 he went into private practice, and died in 1975 aged 73 years.

A keen author Dr Trumper penned two books about his practice, 'Doctor's Weekend' and 'Country Practice'. These were published under the pseudonym of Hubert Bagster, as was 'The Life of a Country Doctor'. At one stage he wrote a column 'Gumboot G.P.' each week in the B.M.J. He also assisted Robin Odell the author of 'Exhumation of a Murder'. This was one of the first books on the death of Katherine Armstrong, the wife of Hay solicitor Herbert Rousse Armstrong.

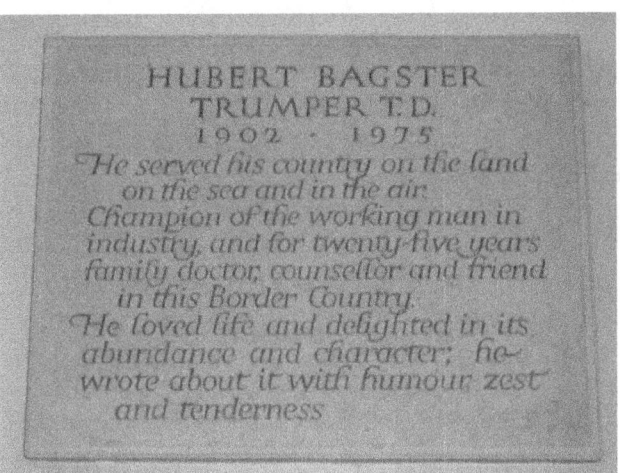

Memorial tablet in Clifford Church.

Hubert married Frances Greener and they had two daughters, Jill and Frances. They rode their ponies into Hay from Clifford each day to attend St Johns School. This was in the building currently a chapel and restaurant opposite the Wheatsheaf public house. The infants were housed in the lower basement room with the senior class upstairs. The girls stabled their ponies at the rear of the 3 Tuns public house, Broad Street.

His son Michael also became a doctor.[70]

WATKINS, Dr Benjamin J.

Piggott's Commercial Directory 1881 lists a Dr Benjamin Watkins practicing in New Street, Hay. He was born in Hay in 1840 and died there in 1927.

WELLINGTON, Edward.

Mr Edward Wellington was an apothecary in Hay but was also referred to as a surgeon. When he died in 1746 his widow Anna moved nearer to her son James in Monmouth.

Anna and James are mentioned in an indenture dated 1st May 1759. This was for the one-year lease of land at Clyfford and Cusop to Richard Morgan, and a piece of land known as 'Poolsound in the Parish of Hay' to Richard Wright.[71]

WILLIAMS, Dr John.

Dr John Williams practised in High Town in 1830 and Back Lane in 1835 but is not listed in any medical directory for 1840. Like many doctors at the time he also appears to have been a farmer. He advertised for a farm of between 60 and 100 acres near Hay, at around £80 a year, between November 1827 and October 1828.[72] Dr Williams died 15 October 1842 aged 46 years, and his wife Mary died 10 March 1851 aged 55 years.

WILSON, Dr Derek.

In 1960 Dr Derek Wilson joined the surgery at Rio Tinto House when he was the only applicant for a job with Dr Hugh Trumper and Dr Wally Wilson. He moved with the surgery to Compton House 1 High Town (now Oxfam) and retired in 1998. He and his wife were officers in the Hay Branch of the St. Johns Ambulance Brigade.

Dr Wilson was one of four G.P.'s who were asked by the B.M.J. to look into the influence of television perceptions on patients concerns about their health. This report was commissioned in response to the big increase in demand for G.P. services in the early 1960's.[73]

WILSON, Dr Walter (Wally).

Dr Walter Wilson was the senior partner of a team of G.P.s in Compton House 1 High Town after the practice moved from Rio Tinto House in 1960.

WOODCOCK, Dr George.

Dr Woodcock was the surgeon who was called to the inquest of Elizabeth Whitford of Brilley in 1848. She died from head wounds inflicted by her partner Thomas Whitford.[74]

In January the following year Dr Woodcock married Mary Anthony at Hanover Square London.[75] They decided to live in London and in 1850 he sold the furniture from his house in Oxford Terrace. Items included country horse saddles, gig harness, surgical instruments, drugs and wine.[76]

As part of settling his affairs in Hay Dr Woodcock took Jason Price to court in June 1850 for non-payment of a bill for £12.11s.6d. This was for journeys and medicine supplied to Price and his wife. Dr Woodcock had attended Mrs Price in June 1849 for inflammation of the lungs. After bleeding her and supplying medicines he attended every day for 10 days.

During this time he noted the condition of Price who had sciatica. Dr Woodcock said he had a machine that would help him. Subsequently Dr

Woodcock attended 26 times at 5s a journey and provided the use of a galvanising machine at 3s a time.

In court Price's defence was that a Mr Lloyd and staff at Hereford Infirmary had declared his sciatica incurable and the galvanising had not improved it. Price disputed that all the visits to himself and his wife were necessary, a view supported by Dr Francis Trumper. Moreover Price had stated to Dr Woodcock that he was a poor man and could not afford the treatment. In response Dr Woodcock had said he would wait two years for payment.

The judge dismissed the action as Dr Woodcock had agreed to a delay for two years but stated Price would need to pay at least a portion of the bill at that time.

Non-Practicing Doctors.

On retiring a number of medical men came to live, or inherited properties, in the Hay area. There is no evidence that they set up medical practices in the town.

BRODBELT, Dr Francis Rigby.

Dr Francis Brodbelt senior (9.10.1746 - 9.12.1795) was a doctor in Jamaica. He qualified in Edinburgh in 1767[77] and to keep ties to his homeland he subscribed to the Caledonian Mercury for many years, as did his son.[78] He married Ann Gardner Penoyre (1.1.1751 - 6.9.1827) of the family at The Moor, Clifford.

Through this connection the Brodbelt family, especially the children, spent considerable holiday time at The Moor. It was the home of Ann's father Thomas Penoyre and then his brother, her uncle, Edmund.

The doctors were important individuals on the island. Like his junior partner, Dr Lee, Dr Brodbelt acquired a large fortune in his practice in Spanish Town. A later partner of Dr Lee, Sir Michael Clare, went on to became Knight member of the Honourable Council and Provincial Grand Master of Freemasons in the Island.

The Robys inscription in St Catherine Cathedral reads:

SACRED TO THE MEMORY OF FRANCIS RIGBY BRODBELT ESQRE. M D WHO IN HIS PASSAGE THRO' THIS PROBATIONARY STATE WAS EMINENTLY DISTINGUISHED FOR PURITY OF SENTIMENT, INTEGRETY OF LIFE AND THE EXEMPLARY DISCHARGE OF EVERY RELATIVE AND SOCIAL DUTY AND WAS EQUALLY RESPECTED AND BELOVED AS A PHYSICIAN AND AS A MAN. HE WAS BORN OCTOBER 9TH 1746; AND DIED DECEMBER 9TH 1795. THIS MONUMENT WAS ERECTED BY HIS SON FRANCIS RIGBY BRODBELT 1799.

BRODBELT, Dr Francis Rigby.

Dr Francis Brodbelt junior (often seen with the additional names Stallard Penoyre) was born on 25 January 1771 and went into practice with his father in Spanish Town Jamaica in 1796.

In 1794, while he was still in England qualifying in medicine, he was the author of a paper entitled 'Case of Disposition of Mercury upon the Bones'.[79] For this he was awarded the silver medal of the Medical Society of Edinburgh on 23 February 1795.

The following year the Annals of Medicine reported on a letter he wrote to 'Dr Duncan'. In it he explained his findings on the gas in the airbladder of a swordfish he caught on the way back to Jamaica. His examination proved that it was oxygen.[80]

A prominent citizen of the island he became a member of the Privy Council of Jamaica. On the 25 July 1803 he married his cousin Frances Gardiner Millward (born 1786) in Spanish Town. On his retirement Dr Brodbelt returned to Britain and settled at Batheaston Villa, Bath.

Dr Brodbelt had been a frequent visitor to his uncle's house The Moor all his life. A Game Licence was issued to him there in 1795. In 1824 he inherited The Moor on the death of his uncle Edmund Stallard. A condition of the inheritance was that he adopted the surname Stallard Penoyre.

Dr Brodbelt had been involved in the extensive rebuild of The Moor from 1822 on behalf of Edmund. In his three years of ownership from 1824 he made alterations to the garden, and also built the tower that is still in existence, although sadly the mansion is gone.

The Jamaican climate had affected Dr Brodbelt's health, and he died of a 'fit of apoplexy at his gate' i.e. a stroke, after a day's shooting on the 29 January 1827, aged 56 years. His death certificate records his death was at Whaplode, Lincolnshire.

His only legitimate child Anna Maria Napleton (born 1804) married the Rev. John Leyson, vicar of Clifford until his death in 1844. From their marriage in 1830 the couple used only the surnames Stallard Penoyre in accordance with Dr Brodbelt's will.[81] Their daughter Maria married the Rev. William T. Napleton Penoyre in 1846.[82]

The Moor was originally in Clifford parish but in 1853 this was split and The Moor became part of the new parish of Hardwicke. Hardwicke Church was endowed by the Penoyre family. Dr Brodbelt's memorial is in Clifford Church,[83] but the east window of Hardwicke Church is also a memorial to him.[84]

Dr Brodbelt had three illegitimate children, all of whom received equal shares in his will. (Possibly a house each in London).

CLUTTERBUCK, Dr.

An advertisement in the Hereford Journal in November 1858 stated that Dr Clutterbuck of London was resuming his practice in his residence at Middlewood, near Hay. No other details known.

HOBSON, Dr Lewis John.

Dr Hobson was 58 years of age in 1911 and staying at the Wye Temperance Hotel, 10 Castle Street, probably on holiday. In 1874 he was in India at the Grand Durbar in Baroda, so may have served in the army. In the late 1870's he established a practice in Harrogate where he was medical officer to the Royal Northern Sea Bathing Infirmary from 1879 to 1891.

HOPE, Dr James Edwin.

When Dr Hope was born in 1844 his parents John and Mary lived at 1A Bear Street, a grocery shop and bakery. His father owned two or three houses in the street and the family later lived at no. 13. By 1861 his father was a builder and cabinet maker.

Dr Hope and his ten siblings were home schooled. After working as a clerk for Griffiths the solicitors he trained at St Bartholomew's Medical School and qualified as a doctor three months before his 21st birthday.

Dr Hope became the 1st Commissioner of Public Health in Western Australia and died on the 21 November 1918. (see pages 145-6).

HOWORTH, Col. Humphrey.

Col. Humphrey Howorth was born in Gladestry in 1749, the son of Sir Humphrey Howorth of Maeslough. Growing into a dissolute young man, strained family finances forced him to join the Honourable East India Company in 1777. He was an assistant surgeon in Bengal in 1778, surgeon in 1781, on furlough in 1785, and discharged by 1793.

During his career in India Col. Howarth acquired £40,000 through the opium trade and proceeded to spend it lavishly in London during the rest of his life. He is buried in Cusop churchyard.

LEWES, Dr Hugh Aythan

Dr Lewes was a surgeon who lived in Broad Street Leominster.[85] He owned Llangwatham House and Llangwatham Mill in Cusop Dingle but there is no indication that he had a practice in Hay.

PHILLIPS, Dr Thomas.

Dr Phillips was born in 1761 and lived his childhood in the family home at Llandegley in Radnorshire. In his teens he was apprenticed to an apothecary in Hay but before he was 20 years of age he went to London. There he studied medicine under the greatest anatomist of his day John Hunter.

After service in the Royal Navy Dr Phillips went to India as a surgeon in the artillery for the Honourable East India Company.

On the 24 January 1800 he married Althea Edwards, the daughter of the Vicar of Cusop, Edward Edwards. On his return to India he made a fortune as a surgeon at Arldleny, Bengal with The Company. In 1817 he returned to England and until his death in 1851 concentrated on the furtherance of education in Wales, including the founding of Llandovery College.

At the time of his death he lived in Brunswick Square London but he was a frequent visitor to Hay. It is not known if he practiced medicine in the town but this appears extremely unlikely. He is buried with his wife in plot no.221 St Marys Churchyard, Cusop.

Dr Phillips presented at least four sets of 30 books to the Mechanics Institute library between 1844 and 1848. The institute was housed in Sycamore House, 24 Broad Street, until it closed in the 1980s.[86]

WALLACE, Dr Arthur William.

Dr Wallace was born 5 January 1900 to Arthur and Alice Wallace, and worked as an apprentice dental technician in Edinburgh from 1915-17.

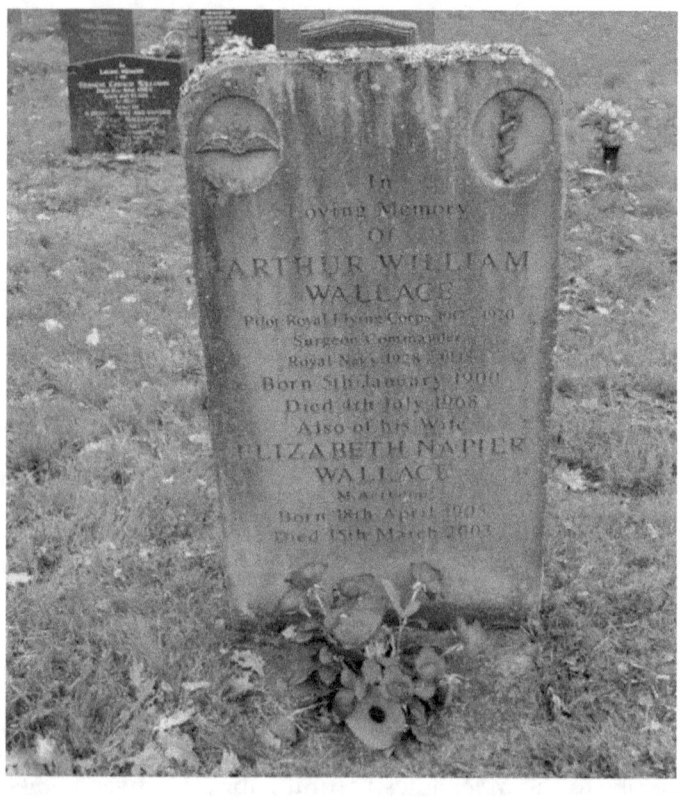

In 1917 he joined the Royal Flying Corps, which became the Royal Air Force in April 1918. He was promoted to sergeant and qualified as a pilot in October 1918. Sgt Wallace was admitted to No. 4

Stationary Hospital Arques near St Omer France for a short time in 1919 when his RAF unit was described as 'Rein Park'.

After the war Dr Wallace qualified in chemistry and physics in the 1920 Royal College of Surgeons Edinburgh Dental Examinations[87] and went on to serve as a Lt Commander, Royal Navy Surgeon, from 1928-1948.

Elizabeth Napier Walden became Mrs Wallace in 1931 and they settled in Gillingham. They are buried together in Cusop churchyard.

WILLIAMS, Dr Hubert.

Dr Williams was the Medical Officer of Health for Glasbury District, and possibly also of Hay, for Hay Board of Guardians. On his death in July 1914 they moved to appoint a separate medical officer for Hay.

Surgery Premises.

With so many doctors in Hay over the years inevitably there were surgeries all over the town at some time or another. Before the formation of the National Health Service (NHS) these were often in or next door to the doctor's own homes. Practices were usually single handed or might be father and son. If a practice was a busy one they might take on an assistant.

After 1948 doctors increasingly started cooperative working, and the NHS actively encouraged this, so now group practices are universal.

Houses have been renumbered and roads renamed but most can be identified. Inevitably the following dates are approximate.

- 25 Broad Street - called Wye Bridge Street before 1850.

Dr E. Proctor – before 1830.
Dr Herbert Proctor – for 50 years including between 1820-61.

- Castle Street.

Dr Henry Caple – there in 1840 but not in 1841.

- Church Street.

Dr Joseph Thomas – from at least 1840 to 1844.

- 3 Church Street.

Dr James Watkins Price Lyde – 1868.

- 7 Church Street

Dr Nicholas Hathaway – 1835 (see Rio Tinto House).

- 66? Church Street.

Dr Francis Robert Trumper – from 1851-61.

- 6 Brooke Street.

Dr Francis Robert Trumper – 1868.

- Pemberton House - also known as 9 Bull Ring.

Dr Linton Bogle – 1868.
Dr Charles Clowson – 1871 to 1880.
Dr Edward A. Appleby – 1881.
Dr Robert John Shepherd – 1891 to at least 1895, then 1912 until he left Hay in 1919.
Dr George W. Featherstone – 1901.
Dr Lewis Daniel Heather – a visitor in 1901 but then the resident doctor until his death in 1912.
Dr Hugh Wybrands Powell – 1919 until 1955.

- Rio Tinto House–13 Broad Street.

Dr Nicholas Hathaway – from 1841 to around 1880.
Dr Molohan – 1880-81.
Dr Thomas S.H. Hincks – 1881 to 1930.
Dr Thomas (Tom) E. Hincks – 1898 to 1932.
Dr L.D. Heather – 1912 – probably as an assistant.
Dr Hugh Wybrands Powell – before moving to Pemberton House in 1919.
Dr Hubert Trumper – 1949 – moving into private practice in 1959.
Dr Derek Wilson – 1950's to 1960.

- Compton House – No.1 High Town (now Oxfam). This replaced 14 Broad Street in 1960.

Dr Walter Wilson.
Dr Francis Trumper.
Dr Derek Wilson.
Dr Maurice (Bill) Anderson.

- 11 Oxford Road - replaced Compton House in 1969.

Dr Maurice (Bill) Anderson.
Dr Alan Crossley.
Dr Nansi Evans.
Dr Mary Hughes.
Dr J.E. Smith.
Dr Derek Wilson.

- HayGarth Surgery, Forrest Road, replaced 11 Oxford Road in 1998.

Conclusion.

Despite its relatively low population almost 50 doctors had surgeries in Hay between 1780 and 1980. This seems an extraordinarily large number for such a small town although how many of them were full-time, part-time or only undertook work for relatively wealthy private patients we will never know.

There is no indication that raging diseases were endemic to justify a large medical workforce. Hay was not a spa town, and there was no major industry other than farming with its scattered population in the towns hinterland.

Undoubtedly this provided a large percentage of their work and the records show how dangerous farming and industry associated with agriculture can be. This was particularly so before the advent of health and safety legislation, machinery guards, and safety inspections.

Working with animals, hand operated machinery and antiquated working practices inevitably meant horrendous accidents. Everyone from housewife to skilled workers to labourers also had to endure hours of backbreaking toil as a normal aspect of rural life.

To care for them took commitment and effort in all hours and all weathers, and the records show that the doctors were up to the task.

The vast majority appear to have displayed a strong work ethic and commitment to the people of Hay. They were up to the challenge and played a prominent role in maintaining the health of the local population.

Notes.
[1] Medical Practice in Radnorshire 40 years ago. *Transactions of the Radnorshire Society.* vol.3. (1933).
[2] https://archives.library.wales/index.php/john-edwin-hope-hay-letters-to-his-son-in-australia.
[3] Foster, Allen, *Foster's Welsh Oddities*, Robert Hale (London, 2015).
[4] Anderson, Maurice, Treatment for the Economy, *B.M.J.* 5531 (9 March 1963) 684.
[5] Anderson, Maurice, Queen Anne's Children, *B.M.J.* 5509 (6 August 1966) 358.
[6] *Hereford Journal* (25 August 1866).
[7] *Hereford Journal* (24 October 1860).
[8] *Hereford Times* (2. November 1867).
[9] *London Gazette* (2 August 1864).
[10] *Robsons* (1840).
[11] *Hereford Journal* (18 May 1842).
[12] *Edinburgh Evening Courant* (3 August 1868).
[13] Obituary *B.M.J.* (September 1883).
[14] http://featherstonhaugh.one-name.net/p245.htm#i7332.
[15] *B.M.J.* (5 January 1929).
[16] *Leominster News and North West Herefordshire & Radnorshire Advertiser* (26 July 1907).
[17] *South Wales Daily News* (12 November 1880).
[18] *The London Gazette* (1 August 1876).
[19] List of Degrees, *Edinburgh Medical Journal*, 31(3) (3 September 1885) 294–295.
[20] *London Evening Standard* (23 August 1875).
[21] *South Wales Daily News* (19 December 1894).
[22] *Brecon County Times* (9 April 1914).
[23] *The London Gazette* (19 December 1922).
[24] *Brecon County Times* (30 November 1900).
[25] Beale, Martin, *The Hay Poisoner*, Robert Hale (London, 1995).
[26] *The London Gazette* (19 February 1943).
[27] *B.M.J.* (17 September 1949).
[28] Hay History Group, *Hay on Wye History Notes* (2018) 39-41.
[29] *Wells Journal* (28 January 1921).

30 *Wells Journal* (2 September 1949).
31 *Brecon County Times* (15 January 1925).
32 *Brecon County Times* (8 October 1914).
33 *Brecon County Times* (29 October 1914).
34 Pugh, E. and T. *Roll of Honour* (2010).
35 *The Cambrian* (25 August 1827).
36 http://Ancestry.com.
37 *Silurian, Cardiff, Merthyr, and Brecon Mercury, and South Wales General Advertiser* (29 March 1851).
38 *Hereford Times* (31 January 1857).
39 Ford, Peter, *Mary Morgan. Victim or Villain of 18th Century Infanticide* (2020).
40 *Banbury Advertiser* (15 October 1885).
41 *The Cardiff and Merthyr Guardian* (9 May 1846).
42 *Kelly's Directory* (1923).
43 *Hereford Journal* (17 December 1845).
44 *Hereford Journal* (19 December 1798).
45 *Hereford Journal* (19 August 1843), *Hereford Times* (10 August 1850).
46 *Hereford Journal* (2 April 1834).
47 *Hereford Journal* (17 March 1852).
48 *Hereford Journal* (12 April 1862).
49 *Hereford Journal* (10 March 1866).
50 *Monmouth Merlin* (1878).
51 *Evening Express* (5 November 1894).
52 *Hereford Journal* (22 April 1857).
53 *South Wales Daily News* (10 March 1866).
54 *Hereford Times* (6 September 1851).
55 *Hereford Journal* (30 May 1860).
56 *Hereford Journal* (24 May 1848).
57 *Hereford Journal* (7 September 1842).
58 *Hereford Journal* (5 January 1848).
59 Fairs, G.L., *The History of the Hay*, Phillimore (Chichester, 1972).
60 *Sun,* London (6 April 1855)
61 *Morning Advertiser* (26 April 1856).
62 *Brecon County Times* (9 June 1866).
63 *Hereford Journal* (12 December 1855).
64 *Hereford Journal* (8 June 1825).

[65] *Provincial Medical and Surgical Journal*, Herefordshire Memorial (4 June 1845) 255-6.
[66] *Hereford Journal* (13 October 1838).
[67] The Health of the Worker in Chromium Plating, *B.M.J.* 1:3668 (25 April 1931) 705–706.
[68] https://www.google.com/url?sa=t&rct=j&q=&esrc=s&source=web&cd=&ved=2ahUKEwixwIi2yc_sAhUUWsAKHcqJBowQFjAAegQIBRAC&url=https%3A%2F%2Fwww.bbc.co.uk%2Fhistory%2Fww2peopleswar%2Fstories%2F54%2Fa2327654.shtml&usg=AOvVaw3d9u6XT89UuWF5Mg11y6Uu
[69] *B.M.J.*, 1(4768) (24 May 1952) 1139.
[70] *B.M.J.*, 1(5956) (1 March 1975) 524.
[71] *National Library of Wales,* File D.D.1, 451.
[72] *Hereford Journal* (7 November 1827, 13th February 1828).
[73] *Birmingham Daily Post* (11 August 1964).
[74] *Hereford Journal* (1 November 1848).
[75] *Cheltenham Chronicle* (26 January 1849).
[76] *Hereford Times* (11 January 1850).
[77] *The Medical Register*, Joseph Johnson (London, 1783).
[78] *Caledonian Mercury* (13 October 1791).
[79] *Memoires of the Medical Society of London* vol.5, p.112.
[80] Extract of a Letter to Dr Duncan, from Dr Brodbelt of Jamaica, Giving an Account of Some Observations and Experiments Made on the Gas Contained in the Air-Bladder of the Swordfish, *Annals of Medicine* (1796) 393-4.
[81] *The London Gazette* (10 December 1830).
[82] *Exeter Flying Post* (20 August 1846).
[83] Mozley, Geraldine. Ed. (Undated) *Letters to Jane from Jamaica 1788-1796*. London, The West India Committee for The Institute of Jamaica.
[84] *Hereford Journal* (10 September 1851).
[85] *Pigott's Directory of Herefordshire* (1835).
[86] *Hereford Journal* (17 December 1851).
[87] *The Scotsman* (15 March 1920).

Appendix 1: Rosa Blanche Williams The Martyr of the Storm

Rosa Williams tragic story demonstrates the grit and perseverance of a woman determined to support her family during difficult times. Dr Tom Hincks attended her inquest to testify to the cause of her death.

Rosa's parents John and Elizabeth Parry were married in 1878 in Hereford, and had 6 children, all girls - Elizabeth (known as Edith), Annie E, Lucy M, Rosa Blanche, Emily May and lastly Margaret Grace born in 1890.

Rosa was only seven when her father John died on 12 November 1893. He was only 44 years old. Rosa's mother Elizabeth stayed on at Llwynpendri, the family farm, in Llowes to bringing up their children.

It is not known where Rosa worked after she left school. A Rosa Blanche Parry is recorded as living in Eaton Bishop, Herefordshire, in 1911. She was a lady's maid. Her birthplace is stated as Gladney Brecon, but the precise location of this is unclear. Possibly the enumerator misheard and should have put Glasbury, the large village near Llowes.

Marriage.

Rosa was 28 years old in 1914 when she scandalised her mother by becoming pregnant before marriage. In such circumstances the normal practice was for girls to marry and/or move out of the area. In Rosa's case she did both.

On the 20 May 1914 Rosa married Richard Thomas Williams in Glasbury Baptist Chapel. Richard had been born ten miles away at Church Barn Farm, Winforton, Herefordshire, in 1889. By 1911 his family were farming at Vedwlyde Farm, Glasbury.

Despite the circumstances of the marriage, it proved to be a good match and Richard proved himself a good husband and a capable farmer. At the time of Rosa's death he was a widely respected district councillor.

Emigration.

Less than a month after their marriage, on the 10 June 1914, Rosa and Richard embarked for Australia on the P&O Steam Navigation Co. ship Berrima. They were two of 521 passengers.

The journey must have been very exciting for the couple from rural Radnorshire. After a short stop at Cape Town the Berrima arrived in Melbourne where Rosa and Richard went on to establish a new life.

The timing of their arrival was fortuitous. Within months the First World War had begun. If they had not left Richard might well have been called up for military service.

Life in Australia.

Rosa and Richard settled in Mildura, Wimmera Province, on the north-west border of Victoria, 340 miles north of Melbourne. This flat semi-arid region had been transformed into a rich horticultural region in 1886 by the first irrigation scheme in Australia. Here they established a successful fruit farm in an area that is now famous for its grape production, as well as almonds, citrus and dried fruit.

The couple had four children in Australia - John William, known as Jack, was born in 1914, Ivor Ernest was born 1915, Doreen was born 1916 and Mary Irene (Renee) was born 20 May 1917.

Rosa and Richard's farm in their adopted homeland Mildura was in an area renowned for its extensive sunshine. Temperatures in the summer months average over 30^0 C and can go over 40^0 C.

Unfortunately Richard had a form of photophobia which made his pupils slow to react and close in bright sunlight. This put him at a high risk of becoming blind. As a result the family decided in 1919 to return to Great Britain.

Return to Radnorshire.

On their return they settled at Pant Farm near Rhulen in Radnorshire, north of Hay. Here Rosa had two more children - David Thomas William was born in 1920 and Richard Allan (always known as Allan) was born 29 February 1924.

Despite Richard's efforts times were hard on the farm. To make ends meet Rosa had to sell her eggs and poultry, and the obvious outlet was the weekly market at Hay. This involved leaving the house early and riding her pony 12 miles up over Llanbedr Hill. Passing through the village of Painscastle Rosa then travelled down through Clyro into Hay, returning home late in the afternoon.

Snowstorm.

On Thursday 22 December 1925 Rosa was up early. She left the farm at 8am to take her chicken to the Hay Dressed Poultry Market.

Late in the afternoon, when it was time to go home after a long day, a snowstorm hit the area. Rosa refused an offer to stay overnight at Clyro, saying 'I'll go. My pony will face it all right'. Riding side saddle she set off home carrying her two paniers either side containing presents for the children.

Halfway home she stopped briefly at the Maesllwch Arms, Painscastle (This has been known variously as the Black Ox, the Roast Ox, and is now the Ox). The landlord William Morgan advised her not to continue due to the conditions, but she insisted on going home because she was still nursing her youngest child.

Rosa left Painscastle at 4.30pm repeating 'I'll go, my pony will face it alright'. Exactly what happened on the hill is imprecise and there are a number of conflicting stories relating to Rosa's death.

Llanbedr Hill.

What is not disputed is that the lane up the hill from Painscastle had high hedges which shielded it from the storm. There was no snow lying there but once out on the top the snow was deep. Tracks show that the pony followed the fence line for a time but then for some reason turned back. Rosa fell off halfway back, and the pony carried on down into some trees where it found shelter.

Rosa was found on her back with her feet through the bottom strands of the barbed wire fence. Her left shoe and stocking were missing and both hands were covered in cuts. Handprints imprinted in the snow on the top strand of the barbed wire showed where she had hauled herself approximately 90 yards back towards the road. Her fish flail was still on her arm. It was here she succumbed to the cold and snow.

The assumption was made at the time that in the snowstorm her horse lost its way. When it stumbled in the deep ridges and dips Rosa must have lost her balance and fallen.

One account thought that she was then dragged along with one foot still in a stirrup. When she became free she found her foot/ankle hurt so much she had difficulty walking. Rosa tried to make her way back to the road by following the fence line but was unable to and froze to death on the hill.

Finding Rosa.

There are a number of differing reports of who found Rosa's body the next day.

- The Brecon and Radnor Express at the time stated that her husband, concerned that she had not returned called his farm workers and others to search for her. They found her pony in the early hours floundering in the deep snow. They searched around and under the snow found her body some 20yards away.

- Another account said her husband was not worried when she did not return home that night, assuming she had stopped at her parent's farm as she had done on occasions before. During the night one of Rosa's daughters (Mary or Renee?) told her father that she could hear someone calling out. Her father soothed her and told her it was just the wind and to go back to sleep. He was not alerted something was wrong until he saw Rosa's pony at the farm gate around 10am the following morning the 23 December. He found Rosa's body after retracing the pony's footprints.
- There is a story that her body was found by her uncle Tom Lloyd of Pentre Farm. He is also said to have retraced the pony's prints, from Pig Tail waterfall.
- A local policeman relates how he discovered Rosa's body, and a legend has grown up about him. It was said that the experience affected him so profoundly that he went off sick ,and subsequently was declared unfit to continue and left the force.

Regardless of who actually found Rosa it was only after an extensive search by numerous people from the neighbourhood that she was found later that day. She was lying on her back with her basket still on her arm. The police took her body to Ireland House, the nearby keeper's cottage, and later it was taken down to Rhulen on a makeshift sledge.

Policeman's Account.

A Radnorshire policeman, Lewis Houghton Williams, has left an eye-witness account of the search. He was around 21 years of age at the time and recorded his memories of the event in his later years.

Lewis was suffering a heavy cold when he heard that Rosa was missing. The doctor advised him to stay in bed, but he insisted on joining the search and he and Sergeant Bailey set out on borrowed horses. While it has been said this was while the storm was still raging, he said in his memoires that they went out searching at 8am staying out until 7pm that day. They found Rosa's body frozen to death on the hill.

From marks in the snow they saw that she had fallen from her pony and been dragged parallel along a barbed wire fence lacerating her legs. The pony was nowhere to be seen.

Lewis guarded the body while a sledge was prepared, and Rosa's body was then transported down to Glasbury. Lewis did not accompany the sledge.

Subsequently Lewis was put on sick leave for three months due to a 'strained heart' and a kidney infection, the effects of his exposure to the elements that day. Eventually he had to resign from the force for ill health reasons, although in the end he lived to be 91.

The Inquest.

Rosa's inquest recorded she left for market at 8am Tuesday 22nd December and that it was not until 10am the following day the alarm was raised. Dr Hincks reported that her ankle was swollen and she would not have been able to walk on it but it did not appear broken. In his view Rosa died 'due to syncope following exposure'.

With hindsight it is possible to speculate that Rosa may have broken the bones in the middle part of her foot – a Lisfranc fracture. This particular injury occurs to cavalrymen who had been thrown from their horse and dragged along the ground with one foot caught in a stirrup. The pressure of the stirrup against the sole of the foot while the toes are still caught cause a fracture dislocation of the mid foot.

If Rosa fell off her pony and was dragged this may have happened to her. It would account for her clinging to the fence for support while trying to go back down the hill to shelter. The injury would be easily overlooked if the foot and ankle were swollen, and without the benefit of X-rays.

Major Walter de Winton's gamekeeper William Price said he had known the hill for 25 years and in his opinion it was impassable that night. He suspected the horse would have turned back by itself when it reached the crest of the hill.

Rosa is buried in the graveyard at the chapel in Painscastle. Her youngest grandchild Richard, aged just one year old, is buried near her. Rosa was only 39 years old.

A large memorial stone records the bleak exposed spot where her body was found on Llanbedr Hill.

Aftermath.

Richard's eldest son Jack was initially told only his mother had 'been lost on Llanbedr Hill' and spent all the next day looking for her before realising she had died. The experience affected him deeply.

The earliest memory of Richard Allen her youngest son is of everyone crying.

After her death Rosa's two eldest children Jack and Ivor stayed on at the farm as they were old enough to work, but the other children were dispersed among relatives. The youngest Richard Allan went to live with an aunt in Kent. Here his aunt said as his father was called Richard he would be known as Allan.

He had a joyless existence until his father remarried in 1933 and he was able to return home to a loving family.

The original Llwynpendri farmhouse where Rosa was born was demolished in the 1950's. It was said that the end wall was unsafe as a consequence of the bombs that fell on the nearby Begyn Hills during the Second World War. All that remains to be seen is the stone step from the threshold to the front entrance embedded amongst the rubble in the middle of the current farmyard.

Accounts of Rosa's Story.

Basic details of Rosa's story are displayed in the Cheesemarket, Castle Square, Hay on Wye. From these the full story was developed with the assistance of:

- Mrs Marion Lally, Rosa's granddaughter.
- Mrs Joan Barnes recording of her father Constable Bailey's reminiscences.
- The reprint in *Haywire* (February 1998) of the Brecon County Times report of the inquest 28 December 1925 into the 'Victim of Storm'.
- Two newspaper articles referring to Rosa.
    - King, Lily, Policeman who risked his health in the search for Rosa, the Martyr of the Storm. *Brecon and Radnor Express* (15 September 2017).
    - Lawson, Gareth, Walk by Tragic Memorial. *Hereford Times* (2014).

Appendix 2: Alice Agnes de Winton

"Mrs Richard de Winton, wife of Major de Winton, who is now at the front, left Laurel Cottage, Hay, on Tuesday, to take up the appointment of superintendent nurse on a Red Cross hospital train with our Expeditionary Force in France. The train is equipped with 500 beds and Mrs de Winton will have some 30 nurses under her. She has had experience of this work in South Africa."
Brecon County Times 5 November 1914.

Alice Agatha Cautley Higgs was born in 1871 at Helmsley, Oswaldkirk, Yorkshire. Her father Edward Hood Higgs was curate of Sutton in the Forrest, married to Frances Julia. Alice had three older siblings, brother Edward C. and a sister Julia Mary born in Sussex, and another brother George C. possibly born in India. Her younger siblings Catherine E.C. and Winifred J.C. were born in Yorkshire.

By 1891 her sister Julia had become principal of a lady's college in Brighton. Her mother Frances was a school help and Alice was also there as a governess.

Nursing.

By now Alice was in her 20's and she decided to train as a nurse. This would have taken at least three years but we have no details of where or when she undertook her nursing training.

There is no record of any military connection in Alice's family but the national patriotism that occurred around the start of the Boer War may have influenced her decision to volunteer as a member of the Army Nursing Service on the 29 January 1900.

Princess Helena the third daughter and fifth child of Queen Victoria became Princess Christian of Schleswig-Holstein on her marriage. Princess Christian had a strong interest in nursing and had agreed to the first President of the British Nursing Association in 1892. In 1897 she founded the Army Nursing Service Reserve.

Recruits were required to be between 25 and 35 years of age, of good character, and have had three years of training and general nursing service before they were eligible to join.

Alice served in South Africa during the 2nd Boer War 1899-1902. We know she was at 12 Stationary Hospital Wakkerstroom (Ladysmith) for a time. This had 150 beds and was opened on the 7 Sept 1900 and closed 31 May 1902. For her service Alice was issued with the Kings South Africa Medal.

Marriage.

In 1902 she married Richard Stretton de Winton in Banbury, Oxfordshire. Richard was a Brevet Major in the Royal Artillery and had been in charge of a pom-pom section in South Africa.

Richard was born 17 December 1869 in New Edinburgh, Russell District, Ontario. His father Major-General Francis Walter de Winton was on a diplomatic attachment. He was the second son of Walter de Winton of Maesllwch Castle.

Some records have Richard being born in 1870 at Woolwich in Kent but this may have been a device to establish his British nationality. He was commissioned into the Royal Garrison Artillery in 1889.

'The wedding took place last week, at St. Mary's, Warkworth, of Major Richard Stretton de Winton (only surviving son of the late Sir Francis de Winton) and Miss Alice Agatha Cautley Higgs, who for two arid a-half years nursed in South African military hospitals as a member of the Army Nursing Service Reserve. The bridegroom, who is in the Garrison Artillery, also served in South Africa, and was on special duty with a pom-pom from August, 1899, until quite recently. The bride was given away. by her father, and Captain Dudley du Chair acted as best man. A reception was subsequently held by Mrs Higgs at Oyerthorpe House, lent for the occasion.by Mr. and Mrs. J. R Blacklock, after which the 'bride and bridegroom left for The Pentre, South Wales, where the early days of the honey-moon will be spent.'
British Journal of Nursing 23 September 1902

On her marriage Alice resigned from the nursing service, and as the wife of a serving officer she travelled with her husband on deployment. In 1911 they were at Fort Ricasoli, Malta.

The electoral registers for Penryn, Cornwall in 1912, 1914 and 1915 show them living at 12 Gyllyngvase Terrance, Falmouth although this may have been their UK address while serving abroad. At the outbreak of the First World War Richard was posted to the front.

Richard's parents had retired to Llanstephan House, Llyswen, so it seems highly likely Alice would have visited the Hay area at some stage.

Red Cross Service.

By 1914 Richard's parents were deceased but Richard's older sister Violet May de Winton had moved into Laurel Cottage, Church Street, Hay. Alice stayed there temporarily following her husband's posting abroad, prior to her taking up nursing duties again.

In 1902 the Army Nursing Service had been reformed as the Queen Alexandra Imperial Medical Nursing Service (QAIMNS), with Queen Alexandra as President. Alice had resigned on her marriage so did not transfer to the new organisation.

At the outbreak of the First World War the number of nurses in the QAIMNS was only around 297 serving sisters, as selection was so rigorous. Of these only 44 nurses had served in the Boer War, and just 37 had the Boer War ribbon, like Alice, and subsequently went on the serve in the First World War.

To overcome the stringent recruitment criteria in the regular service a QAIMNS Reserve was formed. This recruited large numbers of qualified nurses on short term contracts. While Alice could have been one of these, initially she is only recorded as being in the Red Cross, despite her war experience in South Africa.

The British Red Cross and Order of St John of Jerusalem came together on the 24 August 1914 to form a Joint War Committee. They are well known for the creation of Voluntary Aid Detachments (VADs), for which they recruited and trained large numbers of men and women to support the qualified nursing staff. Very quickly the individual members themselves became known as VAD's.

The Brecon County Times report said that Alice left Laurel Cottage in November 1914 to take charge of a Red Cross Hospital Train.

The No 11 Ambulance Train was provided by the Red Cross. It consisted of 3rd Class carriages modified to hold around 500 stretcher cases. Initially this train appears to have been staffed by 11 Red Cross Nurses, although later this was increased to 30, with Alice de Winton as the sister in charge/matron. Life on the trains was very hard and intense.

'I had an interesting piece of work the other day in taking a party of patients who were evacuated,' i.e., discharged to England. It is the great wish of every patient to be marked for Blighty.' Most of them are on stretchers, but are in a very differentiate from when they came to us." After describing an ambulance train-a " wonderful affair, "staffed with doctors and trained nurses............". Dr. Farran says :- " When we arrived, our stretcher-cases were gently lifted from the ambulances and then carried into place in the coach. The ward looks like a cabin on a ship, with the stretchers hung in four tiers on each side-a broad 'passage between them. The walking cases are put into what look like ordinary first-class coaches."
British Journal of Nursing October 21 1916.

Alice saw service with the Red Cross from 25 November 1914 until 25 October 1916 in the TN (Trained Nurse?) Department.

Wimereux.

On the 5 December 1914 she was sent on active service, to Lady Hadfield's Anglo-American Hospital, Wimereux.

A number of hospitals were built and named after the people who financed them, although they were supervised by the military authorities. This would have been Alice's base as matrons did not travel in the ambulance trains themselves.

Alice must have shown her administrative as well as nursing skills as few months later:

> *'Mrs de Winton has been appointed matron of No 2 Hospital Rouen.'*
> British Journal of Nursing March 27 1915.

No.2 British Red Cross Hospital Rouen was opened in September 1914 for British Officers in the Grande Seminare. Rouen was a major centre for the Red Cross. Not only was their ambulance train based there but it also had their hospital and one of its five main stores in France.

The official war diary of Miss Maud McCarthy Matron-in-Chief British Expeditionary Force, France and Flanders makes interesting reference to No.2.

On the 14 March 1915 Matron McCarthy received a message from the matron of No.2 saying the situation was bad and could she come. At the same time she was given a report from Miss Fletcher the matron of the British Red Cross in France who had visited the hospital that day. In her view the staff were in mutiny over the arrival of a new matron and sisters.

On the 15th Matron McCarthy spent most of the day at No.2 and found a state of utter chaos. No one seemed to be in charge and as a consequence there was no system to anything. All staff appearing to do just what they wanted, how they wanted. The main cause of the dissatisfaction appeared to be a new matron had arrived and not been tactful about the hospitals chaotic working.

Matron McCarthy immediately transferred five staff out of the hospital, indicated where changes had to be made, and arranged to return the next day. (A fortnight later she had the five removed nurses sent back to England rather than be redeployed in France.)

Her visit the next day, the 16th, was short. In her view the whole hospital needed reorganising, and she felt the new matron was more than capable of doing that, providing she was tactful.

On the 22 April there is confirmation that this new matron was Alice. She was specifically named as the matron in charge when she forwarded a report on the disturbances to Matron McCarthy.

That Alice was successful in her endeavours at No.2 is indicated by the following:

MENTIONED IN DESPATCHES.
The following are included in the list of names brought to the notice by Sir John French for gallant and distinguished service in the field.
British Red Cross Society Mrs A de Winton.
British Journal of Nursing 8 January 1916.

This was rapidly followed by:

British Red Cross Society
Award of Royal Red Cross First Class to Miss A de Winton
British Journal of Nursing 14 January 1916.

Despite this mention of a First Class Award, Alice was actually gazetted as a matron who was presented with a Royal Red Cross Second Class award by the king at Buckingham Palace on the 19 February.

FETING MRS. DE WINTON
'Mrs. De Winton, Matron of No. 2 Hospital, Rouen,
who has been decorated with the R.R.C., has been entertained at dinner by the Sisters to commemorate the honour. The decorations were carried out in the loyal colours of red, white and blue. They presented Mrs. De Winton with a cut glass and silver liqueur set, as a memento of the occasion.'
British Journal of Nursing January 29 1916.

Home Service.

By early 1917 Alice was home in blighty and on the 28 February she was posted to the Military Hospital Woolwich to train in the duties of a matron. On 10 March 1917 she received her draft to take up a post as matron at the Offices Convalescent Hospital, Eaton Hall and Howarden Castle Chester.

All that is known of her service there was a period of leave in Paris to see her husband from 22 October to 5 November 1918. Her application for leave was granted on the 17 October providing she obtained a passport and submitted verification of her husband's leave approval.

Alice stayed at the hospital in Chester until she retired to The Chalet, Seaford, Sussex on the 8 December 1919. Her husband had retired 12 September 1919 from The Fort, Newhaven.

The Duke of York presented Alice with a Royal Red Cross First Class Award at Buckingham Palace on the 20 July 1920.

It is interesting that while she was known as matron in the Red Cross no mention was made of this rank when she was gazetted although everyone else had their rank described.

Alice was awarded the Victory Medal, British War Medal, and 1915 Star as well as the Royal Red Cross medal for exceptional military nursing service. She was entitled to use the initials ARRC (Associate Royal Red Cross) after her name. In addition to war medals she was also awarded a Distinguished Conduct Medal.

Alice died in the autumn of 1943 in Hammersmith aged 72 years.

References

Anonymous, Medical Practice in Radnorshire Forty years ago, in the *Radnorshire Society Transactions* Vol III (1933).

Beales, Martin, *The Hay Poisoner,* CPI Group Ltd. (1995).

Bennett, David, *Local History in the Pubs and Inns of Hay* (Lulu, 2015).

Bowen, H.V., ed., *A New History of Wales. Myths and Realities in Welsh History.* Llandysul, Gomer (2011).

British Journal of Nursing, various dates http://www.rcnarchives.rcn.org.

Chuinard, E.G., A Medical Mystery at Fort Clatsop, in Saindon, R.A. ed. *Expeditions into the World of Lewis and Clark,* vol. 2. Lewis and Clark Trail Heritage Foundation Inc., Great Falls MT (2003).

Cule, J., *Wales and Medicine,* British Society for the History of Medicine (1975).

Davies, D., *The Roads and Bridges of the Usk Valley above Brecon* (1967).

Davies, John, *A History of Wales.* Penguin (1990).

Deary, T. and Brown, M., *Horrible Histories Measly Middle Ages,* Scholastic (London, 1996).

Fairs, G.L., *A History of Hay.* Phillimore (Chichester, 1972).

Fairs, G.L., *Annals of a Parish. A Short History of Hay on Wye,* Fairs (Hay on Wye, 1994).

Gerald of Wales, *The Journey through Wales and The Description of Wales,* trans. by Lewis Thorpe, Penguin Books (1978).

Gies, Joseph and Frances, *Life in a Medieval Castle*, Harper and Row (New York, 2015).

Grant, J., Article on the Bailey Walk, *Grants Guide to Hay* (1890).

Hay Millennium Society, *Nobody has heard of Hay*. Logaston Press (2002).

Hereford Journal, Adverts for Quacks (1811).

Hoffmann, David, *Welsh Herbal Medicine,* Abercastle Publications (1978).

Howse, W.H., *Radnorshire,* (1949), reprinted for the Radnorshire Society by the Scolar Press (1973).

Howse, W.H., Finds Made in an Old House at Presteigne, in *The Transactions of the Radnorshire Society*, vol. XXXI (1961) 32.

Jones, Peter, *Quid Pro Quo. What the Romans really gave the English language*, Atlantic Books (London, 2016).

Leather, E.M., *The Folk-Lore of Herefordshire*, Jakeman and Carver (1912), reprinted by Lapridge Publications (1991).

Llangottock Local History Society, Survey by Llangottock Local History Society 1958-60 in *Brycheiniog,* vol. 7 (1961) 138.

Maddox, W.C., Some Radnorshire Epitaphs in *Radnorshire Society Transactions,* vol. XXXV (1965) 58-65.

Michael, Pamela, *Public Health in Wales* 1800-2000, A brief history (2008).

http://www.wales.nhs.uk/documents/090203history publichealthen[1].pdf.

Mozley, Geraldine, *Letters to Jane from Jamaica 1788-1796*, The West India Committee (London,1938).

Mount, Toni, *Dragon's Blood and Willow Bark. The Mysteries of Medieval Medicine*, Amberley Publishing (Stroud, 2015).

National Archives Kew, various military and service records https://www.nak.org.

National Archives, *War Diary: Matron-in-Chief British Expeditionary Force, France and Flanders*. WO95/3988-91. http://www.scarletfinders.co.uk.

Nicholls, A.J., *Historic Directory of Hay*, Lulu (2014)

Nicholls, A.J., *The Lords of the Manor of Hay*. Lulu (2015).

Palmer, Roy, *Folklore of Radnorshire*, Logaston Press (2001).

Plomer, William, ed. *Kilvert's Diary 1870 – 1879,* Vintage Books (London, 1938).

Pugh, Eric and Pugh, Tim, *To The Fallen*, Hay and District Branch of the Royal British Legion (2010).

Sarkey, J., *The Medicine Tree. Traditional Healing in Wales from pre-history to the present*, Llanerch Press (Lampeter, 2009).

Stapleton, Edward J. *An Evacuee in the Hay and other stories* (2012).

Suggett, Richard, *A History of Magic and Witchcraft in Wales,* The History Press Ltd. (Stroud, 2008).

Tipper, David, *Stone and Steam in the Black Mountains*, Blorenge Books (Abergavenny, 1975).

Willcox, Phillip, *The Detective-Physician - The Life and Work of Sir Phillip Wilcox 1870 - 1941*. Heinemann Medical Books (1970).

Williams, Dr R., Reflections from a Doctor's Day Book in *The Radnorshire Transactions*, Vol XXVI (1956) 5-9.

Withey, Alun, *Physick and the Family: Health Medicine and Care in Wales 1600-1750* (Manchester, 2011).

Withey, Alun, Was Wales a Medical Backwater? in Bowen, H.V. ed. *A New History of Wales. Myths and Realities in Welsh History*. Gomer (2011).

Ziegler, Phillip, *The Black Death*, Alan Sutton Publishing Ltd. (London, 1969).

Registers and Directories.

Medical Register, (Flint), 1780, Nuffield Library.

Medical Register for the Year 1783, London, Joseph Johnson.

Physicians of Myddfai. *Red Book of Hergest*. Owned by Jesus College, Oxford, Bodleian Library.

Piggotts Commercial Directory, 1830, 1840, 1844, 1858, 1881.

Robsons Commercial Directory London and Western Counties N.E.S. Wales (1840).

Slaters Royal National Commercial Directory Gloucester and N.S. Wales (1839, 1868).

Worrals Directory of South Wales (1875).

Newspapers.
Brecon County Times.
Hereford Journal.
Hereford Times.
Monmouthshire Merlin.
South West Daily News.
Haywire.

Index

Accidents, 58.
Acton, William, 40.
Alcohol, 17, 61-2, 71, 93, 95.
Almshouses, 48-51, 61, 67, 86, 107-8, 182.
Armstrong poisoning, 27, 113, 122, 167, 190.
Arsenic, 25-7, 32, 105, 120, 122, 167.
Bayes, Mr, 25.
Bald's Leechbook, 12.
Board of Guardians, 42, 79, 126-31, 154, 201.
Bradley, Bramwell, 72.
Brecon, 31, 40, 52, 64, 67, 75, 88, 112-14, 116, 136-7, 145, 163, 168, 171, 176-7, 180, 207.
Brecon Road, 44, 50-1, 53, 93-4, 96, 106-8, 124.
Breconshire, 116, 125, 187.
Breconshire Rifles, 153, 162.
Chemists/ pharmacy, 117-124.
Childbirth, 65.
Crown Hotel, 100, 121.
Cusop, 53, 66-7, 80, 89, 92, 95, 99, 106, 108-16, 124-5, 128, 134, 163, 165, 167, 174-5, 19, 198-9, 201.
Dentistry, 102-5.
De Winton, Alice, 111, 220-27.
De Winton, Rev. J.J., 55, 90, 99.
De Winton, Family (various), 99, 111, 216.
Disease, 5-7, 9, 15-6, 21, 24-6, 28-48, 131-2, 136, 152.
  Cholera, 35, 39-41, 43, 81.
  Diphtheria, 26, 44, 78, 132.
  Ergotism, 29.
  Leprosy, 30, 36.

Measles, 46, 78-9, 131.
Plague, 30-34.
Scarlet fever, 45, 78, 82, 131-2, 134-5, 156.
Smallpox, 35, 41-43, 131-3.
Sweating sickness, 34.
Tetanus, 47.
Tuberculosis, 17, 26, 35-8, 84, 137-8.
Typhoid fever, 11, 35, 42-3, 79.
Whooping cough,16, 44-5, 78.
Drainage, 40, 81, 96-8.
Drowning, 60, 67.
Folklore, 6, 10,13, 118.
Friendly Societies, 51-4, 95, 100, 163.
Grwyne Fawr Camp, 165-6.
Hay Union, 79-80, 131, 162, 181, 184-5.
Hay Medical Officers, 35, 52, 66, 69, 82-4, 127.
Hay and Cusop Nursing Association, 108-11, 116, 130, 163.
Herbal, 6-10, 119, 141.
Hermeticists, 21.
Hospitals.
  Isolation, 43, 46-7, 131-6, 164.
  Mid-Wales Lunatic Asylum, 136-7.
  South Wales Sanitorium, 38, 107, 137-8.
  Union House, 126-31.
Inquests, 66, 68, 70-1.
Kilvert, Francis, 6, 17, 19, 25, 37, 45, 51, 103, 155.
Llangattock, 15-6.
Llanigon, 6, 61, 80, 120, 149.
Medical Practitioners – chapter 6.
  Appleby, 83, 146, 150, 184, 203.
  Bogle, 58-64, 68, 70, 126, 146, 151-3, 182-85, 203.

Brodbelt, F.R. senior, 194-5.
Brodbelt, F.R. junior, 195-7.
Bridgewater, 62, 154, 184.
Caple, 80, 154-5, 202.
Clouston, 17, 35, 83, 150, 155-6.
Clutterbuck, 197.
Dickson, 83, 156.
Featherstone, 83, 157, 203.
Giles, 25, 83, 157-8.
Hincks, (Arthur) Cecil, 168-170.
Hincks, Thomas S.H., 64-5, 116, 146, 162-4, 173, 177, 184, 203.
Hincks, Thomas Ernest (Tom), 27, 38, 53, 59, 62, 67, 72, 83-4, 91, 97, 100, 109, 113, 117, 122, 129, 134, 163-8, 173, 179, 185, 203, 209, 215.
Hincks, Others, 168-72.
Hobson, 197.
Hope, 145-6, 198.
Howorth, 198.
Lewes, 199.
Lloyd, 59, 194.
Lyde, 62, 68, 144-7, 155, 174-7, 187, 202.
Phillips, 150, 199.
Powell, 63, 179, 203.
Proctor, 21, 52, 58, 63, 83, 126, 146, 180-2, 202.
Reece, 19, 24, 52, 59, 68-9, 146, 156, 176, 183.
Shepherd, 46, 67, 82-3, 162, 184-5, 203.
Smith, 61, 83, 107, 146-7, 182, 185, 204.
Taylor, H., 185.
Taylor, J.C., 61, 186-7.
Trumper, F.R., 58-9, 63, 68, 146, 155-6, 187-8, 202.
Trumper, H.B., 189-90, 192, 203.

Wallace, 200-1.
Williams, H., 201.
Williams, J., 192.
Williams of Talgarth, 145, 184.
Medieval, 5 et al, 29-30, 33, 76, 79, 85, 93.
Midwifery, 110, 115-7, 137.
Moor, The, 53, 59, 194-7.
Nursing, 72, 105-17, 129, 136-7, 166, 219-27.
Paediatrics/children, 10, 38, 62-7, 78, 127, 135.
Pharmacists, 117-24.
Physicians of Myddfai, 7-9.
Public Health, 75-100.
Public Houses, 93-5, 180.
Rose and Crown, 37, 51, 60, 94, 180.
Sant, Esdras, 122.
Septicaemia, 48.
Suicide, 66-7.
Surgery, 13, 57, 142.
Surgery Premises, 201-204.
Swan Hotel, 37, 71, 93, 103.
Urban District Council, 83, 90, 92, 96, 116, 130-36, 163-4, 184.
Vagrants, 43, 128-32.
Vestry Committees, 79.
Water Supply, 40, 71, 81, 84-92.
Weobley, 18.
Wills, G.S.V., 120.
Williams, Rosa, 71-2, 209-18.
Whishlade, Benjamin, 45-6.
Workhouse, 42, 48, 64, 80, 88, 106, 109, 124-34, 162, 181-82.

Also by the same author.

Mary Morgan.
Victim or Villain of 19th Century Infanticide?

The story of poor Mary Morgan, the servant girl in 'the big house' who becomes pregnant, conceals her pregnancy, and then kills her baby at birth is not unique. Neither is the rapid discovery of the body, the trial and the verdict guilty of murder.

What is so poignant is that just a few miles away there is another young servant girl called Mary. When she becomes pregnant and kills her new-born child, she is sentenced by the same judge to a lesser penalty for only the 'concealment of birth'.

Was Mary Morgan a hapless victim of a harsh social structure where the 'have nots' had few rights? Were their different sentences an indictment of the legal system at the time? What did it say about society?

Who was the father? Was there a conspiracy against one Mary and not the other? Did the judge have an ulterior motive?

Time has not mellowed the horrific details. One Mary was sentenced to two years in goal, the other Mary was hanged. A judicial killing? Which Mary received appropriate justice?

Judge for yourself the case of Mary Morgan, victim or villain.

Available for Amazon.

Fair Rosamund.
Mistress of King Henry II.

Rosamund was the daughter of Walter Clifford, the powerful Marcher lord who usurped Clifford Castle from his overlord. Anxious to curry favour with the king the baron introduced Rosamund to King Henry II.

He is successful beyond his wildest dreams, and his daughter's life is changed forever. 'Fair Rosamund', the noted beauty, is whisked away by the king to his secret palace of Woodstock in Oxfordshire.

There are few verifiable details of the rest of Rosamund's life, but she leaves a myriad of legends and stories about her, including:

She was named after a rose.
She had two children.
She lived in a maze.
The only way in was following a silken cord.
She was poisoned by the evil Queen Eleanor.
Or was it stabbed.
She died very young.

How did these come about? Is there any truth in them? Why is Rosamund the mistress so idolised, but Eleanor the wronged wife so demonised.

This book explores the truth behind the stories, and the myriad of books, poems, plays and pictures depicting this ephemeral heroine.

Available from Amazon.

www.ingramcontent.com/pod-product-compliance
Lightning Source LLC
Chambersburg PA
CBHW072027230526
45466CB00020B/1006